Karim Hachelaf
Med Amine Benzemrane
Ouahiba Kerri

Surgical treatment of osteogenesis imperfecta

Karim Hachelaf
Med Amine Benzemrane
Ouahiba Kerri

Surgical treatment of osteogenesis imperfecta

ScienciaScripts

Imprint
Any brand names and product names mentioned in this book are subject to trademark, brand or patent protection and are trademarks or registered trademarks of their respective holders. The use of brand names, product names, common names, trade names, product descriptions etc. even without a particular marking in this work is in no way to be construed to mean that such names may be regarded as unrestricted in respect of trademark and brand protection legislation and could thus be used by anyone.

Cover image: www.ingimage.com

This book is a translation from the original published under ISBN 978-620-6-71342-5.

Publisher:
Sciencia Scripts
is a trademark of
Dodo Books Indian Ocean Ltd. and OmniScriptum S.R.L publishing group

120 High Road, East Finchley, London, N2 9ED, United Kingdom
Str. Armeneasca 28/1, office 1, Chisinau MD-2012, Republic of Moldova, Europe
Printed at: see last page
ISBN: 978-620-7-67350-6

Copyright © Karim Hachelaf, Med Amine Benzemrane, Ouahiba Kerri
Copyright © 2024 Dodo Books Indian Ocean Ltd. and OmniScriptum S.R.L publishing group

SUMMARY

Osteogenesis imperfecta is a rare pathology characterized by bone fragility, leading to repeated fractures and limb deformities. It is diagnosed biologically, clinically and radiologically.

Genetic research has led to a better understanding of this disease, and the introduction of medical treatment and bisphosphonates have revolutionized its management.

This condition is both constitutional, associating bone fragility with recurrent fractures and skeletal deformity; prolonged immobilization leads to osteopenia, thus aggravating the disease; it is essentially for these reasons that surgery must provide effective protection.

Surgery is an important palliative option in the therapeutic management of this pathology.

Segmental osteosynthesis should be avoided. Since SOFIELD's first publications, surgery using an internal stent has opened the door to the current principles of modern surgery in this pathology.

Internal stent osteosynthesis remains the method of choice. We have moved on from the single nail of SOFIELD to the telescopic nail of BAILEY and DUBOW to meet the principles of complete protection of the long bone during the growth period.

Radiography and technology have led to improvements in osteosynthesis equipment; the BAILEY and DUBOW nails have been extensively modified by various authors to better meet the principles of palliative surgery for this pathology.

Telescopic or sliding pinning is a highly attractive technique for the management of long bone fractures and deformities in osteogenesis imperfecta. It is a simple and inexpensive technique. The different variants of this technique enable the surgeon to adapt the most appropriate set-up to the bone deformities and manifestations. Radiological analysis enables the surgeon to decide on the type of pinning (centromedullary, mixed or subperiosteal) and any associated procedures required to correct deformities or contain a fracture.

Surgery for spinal deformities must be part of the therapeutic arsenal for this disease, to avoid life-threatening respiratory complications in these children.

The success of any surgical procedure depends not only on technical mastery, but also on multidisciplinary management involving paediatricians, rheumatologists, rehabilitation specialists, physiotherapists, psychologists, patients' parents and society as a whole, to name but a few.

Table of contents

I. GENERAL

Osteogenesis imperfecta (OI) is the literary term for unreliable bone production.

It is the only orphan bone disease considered a rare disease by Algerian lawmakers [1].

This disease encompasses a range of bony and extra-bony manifestations of varying severity.

The clinical consequences of **osteogenesis imperfecta** are heterogeneous. They range from pre- and peri-natal death to fractures, deformities, cardiorespiratory disorders, deafness and metabolic disorders.

It's a genetic condition that can only be managed within a multidisciplinary framework.

The advent of medical treatment, led by bisphosphonates (BP), has changed the poor prognosis of this disease.

The principle of correcting deformities and restraining them with an intramedullary stent opened the door to the development of modern intramedullary osteosynthesis techniques. These techniques, such as telescopic nailing and sliding pinning, ensure bone protection during growth.

Today, the effectiveness of palliative surgical techniques depends on multidisciplinary management: rehabilitation, orthopaedic devices, the development of radiology, the quality of anaesthesia and the advent of painkillers and bisphosphonates have transformed the natural evolution and prognosis of this condition.

I.1.   History :

Osteogenesis imperfecta is a pathology known since ancient times [2], [3]. It was observed more than ten centuries before Christ, as witnessed by the bone characteristics of osteogenesis imperfecta found on the bones of a mummy from the Beni-Hassen necropolis near the Nile, discovered in 1907. This mummy was studied by Gray in 1969. It is currently preserved in the Museum of London [4], [5], [6].

In the 7th century, the discovery of a skeleton with a morphology compatible with a variety of deformities due to the disease was reported in the literature [3], [5].

The most famous case of osteogenesis imperfecta was observed in the 11th century. That of the Danish Viking commander IVRAR BENLOS, nicknamed IVRAR THE BONELESS, who invaded England carrying a shield [3], [5].

In 1678, Malebranche first described osteogenesis imperfecta [3], [5].

In 1788, ECKMAN, a Swede, published the case of a subject suffering from the disease with numerous deformities, having had affected children himself [7].

In 1835, LOBSTEIN (Figure N°1), a midwife from Strasbourg, gave a detailed description of this bone fragility, which he called osteopsathyrosis [3], [5].

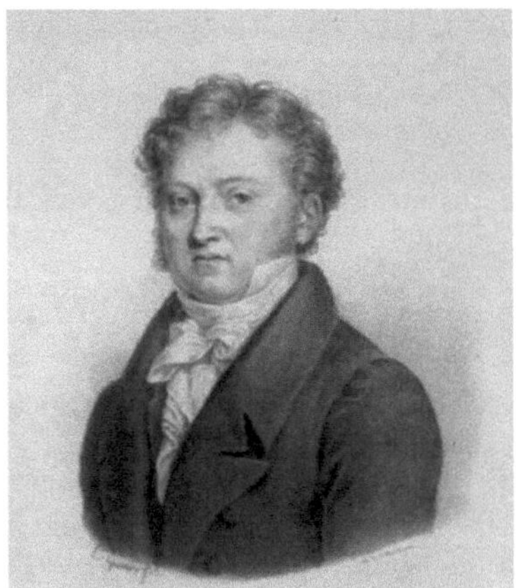

Figure 1: Photo of Mr LOBSTEIN

In 1849, VROLICK distinguished osteogenesis imperfecta from rickets, giving it its current name "osteogenesis imperfecta" [3], [5].

BAUER and KNAGGS were the first to hypothesize that the bone changes of osteogenesis imperfecta were due to osteoblast dysfunction [3], [5].

In 1889, STILLING established the first histological data on the disease [3], [5].

In 1894, PORACK and DURANTE highlighted the predominance of periosteal alterations in ossification disorders, and MOREAU presented his thesis on osteogenesis imperfecta [3], [5].

In 1906, LOOSER made the connection between osteopsathyrosis and osteogenesis imperfecta. He described two forms of osteogenesis imperfecta, depending on the age at which the first fractures occurred and their severity [3], [4], [5] :

- Osteogenesis congenita (severe form with fractures from birth)

- Osteogenesis tarda (less severe fracture occurring after birth)

In the 20th century, EDDOWERS identified the association between osteogenesis imperfecta and blue sclera [3], [4], [5].

In 1918, VANDER HOEVE and DE KLEIN described the association of hereditary nature, bone fragility, deafness and blue sclera with the disease [3], [4], [5].

In 1928, E. APERT proposed the name "glass bone disease" for this illness [3], [4], [5].

In 1933, DANIELUS was the first to make an in utero radiological diagnosis of a pregnant woman whose 8th-month X-ray showed an invisible foetus [3], [4], [5].

The rarity of osteogenesis imperfecta, combined with the diversity of its forms, explains the perplexity of physicians, each of whom has only limited experience. It is only thanks to the gathering of a sufficient number of observations and their classification that knowledge of this pathology has evolved.

The twentieth century was the era of clinical, genetic and pharmacological research. This progress in research made it possible to establish a relatively precise diagnosis and a modern multidisciplinary therapeutic orientation.

The introduction of bisphosphonates by NAGANT and DEVOGLAER [8] in 1984 revolutionized the management of osteogenesis imperfecta.

Genetic and biochemical studies developed over the last 20 years have led to the discovery of new forms of osteogenesis imperfecta, and to the adaptation of modern therapeutics.

Surgery has undergone several periods of development. It went from the idea of aligning the diaphyses and protecting them with a single centromedullary alignment nail "initiated by SOFIELD [9] in 1952", to the current telescopic nail by FASSIER-DUVAL [10] used since the 2000s. During this period, the initial telescopic nail of BAILEY DUBOW [11], used since 1963, was developed. Telescopic pinning according to METAIZEAU [12] was introduced into the surgical arsenal in 1987 for surgery on osteogenesis imperfecta (figure N°02).

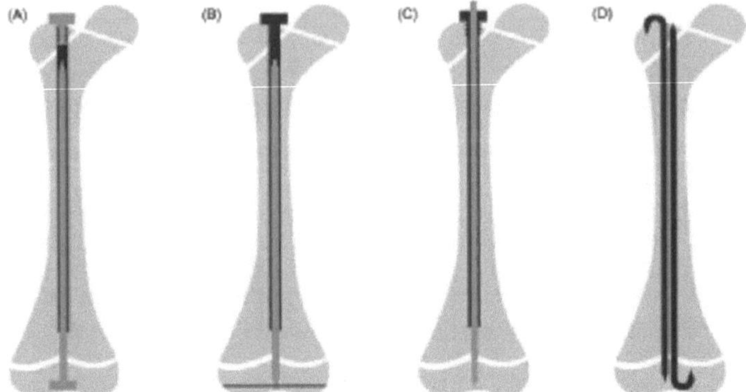

Figure N°02 : *Various centromedullary telescopic osteosynthesis devices: a- Bailley-Dubow nail, b- Tae-Joon Cho et al nail, c- Fassier- Duval nail, e- Métaizeau centromedullary telescopic pinning.*

Thanks to the efforts made in recent years to tackle this rare disease, we can now offer patients appropriate, multidisciplinary care.

I.2.   Definition:

Osteogenesis imperfecta is a mysterious disease. Numerous authors have given it several names found in the literature [13].

- Periosteal dystrophy
- Fragilis or fragilitas ossium
- Osteopsathyrosis idiopathica
- Glass bone disease
- Lobstein's disease
- Vrolik's disease
- Porak and Durante disease
- Fetal rickets
- Hereditary fibrous osteodysplasia
- Osteomalacia congenita
- Osteoporosis fetalis
- Eddowes syndrome
- Van der Hoever syndrome

Osteogenesis imperfecta is a rare hereditary genetic condition characterized by congenital bone fragility associated with low bone mass [14]. This condition results in widespread, diffuse osteoporosis, leading to repeated pathological fractures and bone deformities of varying severity (Figures N°03 and N°04).

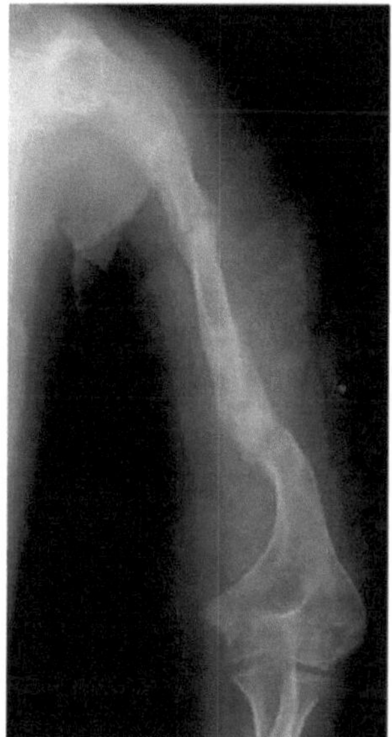

Figure N°03: *Radiograph of a case of humeral osteogenesis imperfecta [personal collection]:*

- *Osteoporosis*
- *Different age fractures*
- *Deformations*

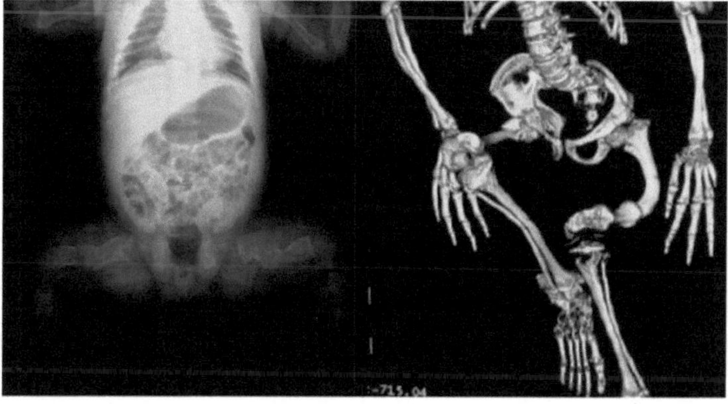

Figure N°04: representative images of some bone manifestations in osteogenesis imperfecta [personal collection].
a- X-ray image of skeletal deformities
b- CT images of skeletal deformities

Osteogenesis imperfecta is a syndrome that groups together a number of hereditary conditions with highly variable clinical manifestations and degrees of presumption. It may be associated with generalized osteoporosis, dentinogenesis disorders, a triangular face, bluish sclerae, often short stature, ligament laxity, excessive sweating, a tendency to bruise, cardiorespiratory disorders, progressive hearing loss, bone pain and fractures occurring without trauma or on the occasion of minor trauma [15].

Osteogenesis imperfecta (osteogenesis imperfecta), or glass bone disease, remains a rare genetic disorder characterized by bone fragility and osteopenia [16], [17].

I.3.   Epidemiology :

It's a rare pathology, considered the only rare bone pathology in Algeria. At present, we have no national epidemiological figures. A rare disease registry is being set up at the Institut National de Santé Publique for 2019.
Osteogenesis imperfecta affects both sexes, with no ethnic predominance.

It is a congenital pathology that can manifest itself ante-, peri- or post-natally. Some mild forms may go undetected and manifest late in life.
The birth prevalence of osteogenesis imperfecta is around 1 per 10,000 to 20,000 births in France, with an incidence of osteogenesis imperfecta of 1-2/10000 [18]. Prevalence in DENMARK is 10.6 per 100,000 people, with an incidence of 15/100,000 births [19], [20].
Prevalence in BRAZIL is 4.0-6.7 per 100,000 births and incidence 4.3 / 1000000 births [21], [22].

The vast majority (90%) of patients with osteogenesis imperfecta have an autosomal dominant mutation [23]. In the last ten years, rare autosomal recessive forms (around 6 to 8% of all cases of osteogenesis imperfecta) have been identified [24]. More recently, Van DIJK et al have shown that 2-4% of osteogenesis imperfecta is X-linked [25].

The expression of the disease varies widely, ranging from moderate forms that often go unnoticed to major lethal perinatal forms.

At present, no national statistics are available. If we refer to the distribution of patients treated at the DOUERA University Hospital, this is a frequent pathology in the center of the country (Figure N°05).

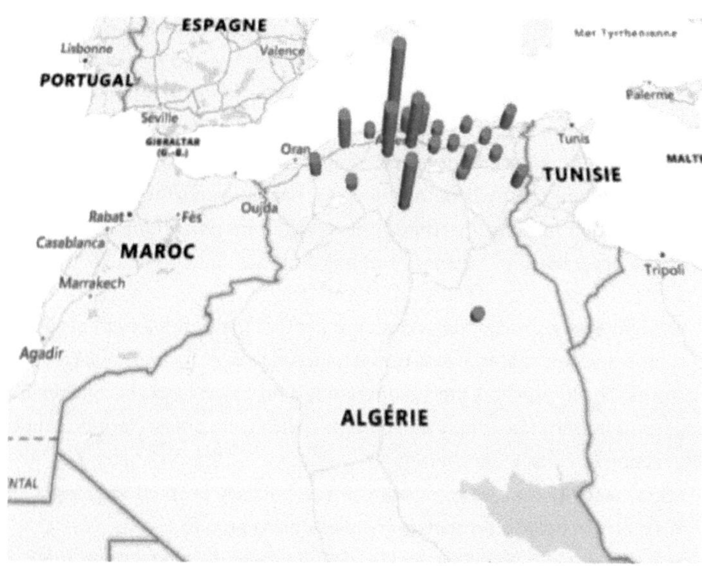

Figure N°05: *Breakdown of national origins of patients treated in the department [personal experience].*
The bars represent the number of patients per wilaya.

II. PROBLEMS

Osteogenesis imperfecta is a mysterious, rare condition characterized by congenital bone fragility. It is genetic in origin. In 90% of cases, it is due to mutations of autosomal dominant transmission, and in 10% of cases, the mutation is of autosomal recessive transmission [26], [27].This disease encompasses a range of bony and extra-bony manifestations of varying severity. Its clinical consequences are heterogeneous, ranging from death to fractures, deformities, blue sclerae, hyperlaxity, respiratory disorders, deafness and metabolic disorders. Fractures occur frequently and repeatedly, following minor trauma.

Bone deformities are secondary to the malleability of bones, which are unable to stretch adjacent muscles and tissues as they grow.

Medical treatment, led by bisphosphonates, has changed the prognosis of this disease. Although medical treatment improves bone densitometry, it does not prevent the occurrence of fractures and deformities.

Segmental osteosynthesis does not protect the entire length of the bone. On the contrary, this material exerts mechanical loads at its ends, which can lead to fractures. This is why it is not recommended for osteosynthesis of fractures in osteogenesis imperfecta. It may be combined with centromedullary protection in the correction of certain deformities.

SOFIELD [9] was the first to introduce centromedullary protection, using a single nail. This nail is unable to protect long bones during growth.

This principle opened the door to the development of modern intramedullary osteosynthesis techniques.

BAILLEY and DUBOW [11] introduced the telescopic nail. This nail consists of two parts, a solid male part sliding into a hollow female part. This sliding principle ensures the protection of long bones during growth. Since then, several improvements have been made to this nail, with the aim of improving its morbidity.

In 1987, with the development of radiology techniques and elastic centromedullary pinning for the treatment of long-bone fractures, METAIZEAU [12] introduced telescopic or sliding centromedullary pinning for the treatment of deformities and fractures in osteogenesis imperfecta. Restraint is provided by two pins. One descends from the proximal epiphysis, the other ascends from the distal epiphysis. These two pins provide protection from one epiphysis to the other. Sliding one on top of the other ensures continuous protection during growth.

Sliding pinning has also undergone modifications; GEORGE FINIDORI [28], [29] has extended the use of this principle by placing pins extra-medullarily, sub-periosteally in severe forms with no possibility of repermeabilizing the diaphyseal shaft.

Telescopic nailing and sliding pinning are only palliative osteosynthesis techniques used to improve the functional prognosis of children with osteogenesis imperfecta. The surgeon has only one role to play in the management of this pathology.

In view of the multitude of surgical techniques listed in the literature, we have chosen the telescopic pinning technique for evaluation and adaptation to our particular health context.

Today, the effectiveness of palliative surgical techniques depends on multidisciplinary management. Post-operative follow-up, preparation of orthopaedic devices, rehabilitation, medical treatment, schooling for children and parental support are all part of a long and complex process. If we want to give patients every chance of reintegrating into society, we need to organize multidisciplinary care.

The public authorities need to get involved in treating this pathology, which poses a public health problem and would be prohibitively expensive to treat abroad.

III. Anatomophysiological reminder:

III.1 The chondro-epiphysis and periosteum :

III.1.1. Chondro-epiphysis/Growth cartilage :

Growth plate (GG) is largely a histological structure interposed between the epiphysis and the diaphysis (Fig. N°06). It contributes essentially to bone length growth. This notion is obsolete, as the CC is not a disc interposed between the epiphysis and the metaphysis. It is an integral part of the epiphysis, with which it forms a mechanical and vascular entity known as the chondro-epiphysis [30].

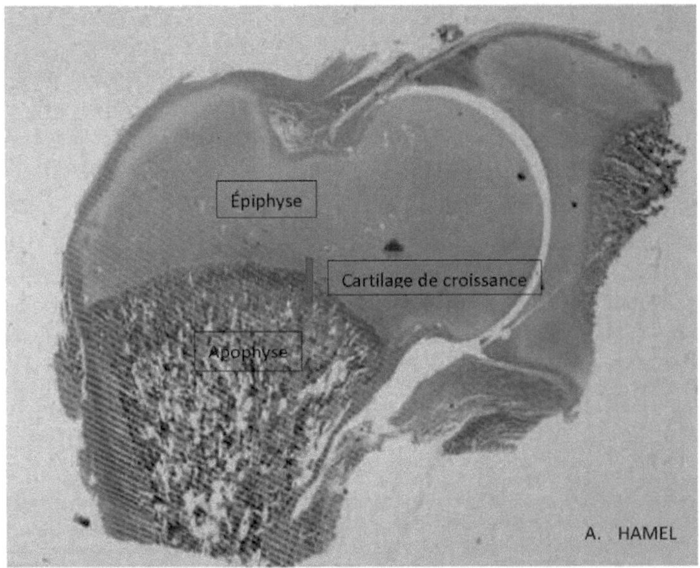

Figure N°06: Superior femoral chondro-epiphysis after A. HAMEL

This entity is made up of an ossification core entirely circumscribed by its growth plate. Growth cartilage is particularly active on the metaphyseal side. It ensures bone growth in length and contributes to its shape. It is completely inseparable from the epiphyseal core [31].

On the metaphyseal side, the junction of the CC with the neoformed bone constitutes a line of fragility, the elective site of epiphyseal detachments. This weak point in the growing bone is compensated for by a collagenous fibrous sleeve at the periphery of the metaphyseal CC. This fibrous sleeve is the perichondral ferrule [32].

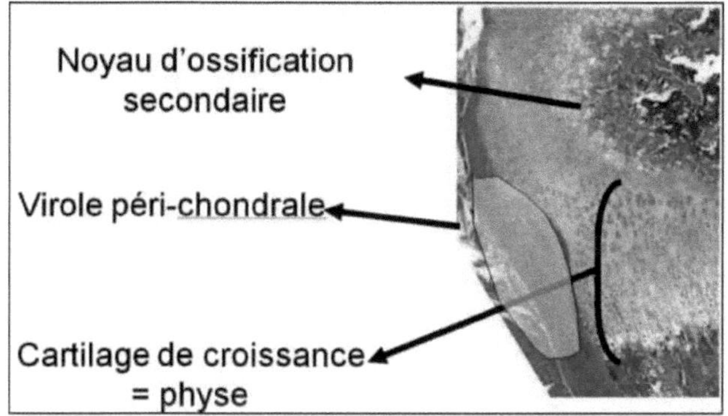

Figure N°07: Histological image of the perichondral shell [28].

The perichondrial ring (Fig. N°07) forms the junction between the chondro-epiphysis and the periosteum. According to the work of Chun [33], it plays a supporting role. The perichondrial ring and chondro-epiphysis together form a biomechanical unit adapted to the physiological constraints of growing bone.

III.1.2. Vascularization of the chondro-epiphysis:

The entire CC is vascularized by vessels of epiphyseal origin (figure N°08 and N°09) and there is a true vascular border between the chondro-epiphysis and the metaphysis [34].

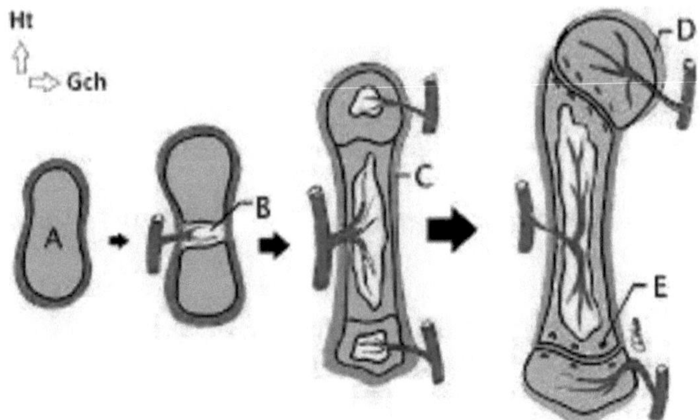

Figure N°08: *development of the metaphyseal vascularization (EMC) :*

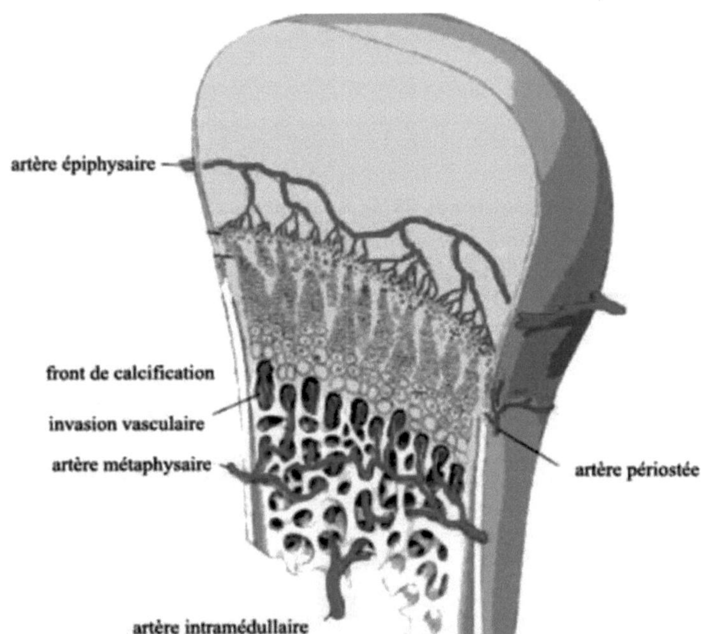

Figure N°09: *vascularization of the chondro-epiphysis (EMC)*

This vascular no-man's-land is located in the degenerative layer at the junction with the neoformed bone (Fig. N°09), i.e. at the epiphyseal detachment line. Thus, even in cases of major displacement, epiphyseal detachment does not compromise chondroepiphyseal vascularization. On the other hand, if an abnormal continuity solution exists in the CC, a definitive communication is formed between the metaphyseal bone and the epiphyseal bone, thus constituting an epiphysiodesis bridge.

The epiphysiodesis bridge is constant for any interruption of the CC. Its consequences vary according to its relative volume and histological nature.

Thus, when the growth CC is crossed by a pin (Fig. N°10), the continuity solution is of the order of a millimeter, and the epiphysiodesis bridge produced is essentially fibrous and thin, constituting a weak mechanical resistance that cannot oppose growth [31].

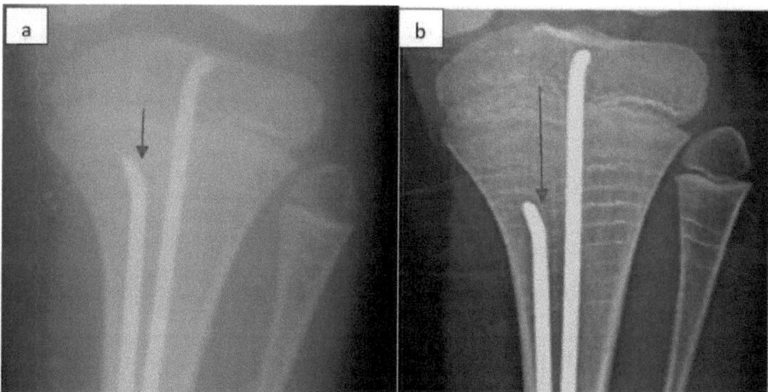

Figure N°10: Continuous activity of the CC crossed by a pin [personal collection] a- Postoperative X-ray b- X-ray at 8 months postoperative

III.1.3. The periosteum:

The periosteum is a fibro-cellular tissue (figure N°11), which plays a biological and mechanical role. It consists of two layers [30]:

A superficial, fibrous layer in contact with the soft tissues. It plays a mechanical role

A deep osteogenic layer. This layer is responsible for the massive production of bone tissue. It is involved in the growth of bone segments and in the consolidation of fractures.

The periosteum is an osteogenic biological membrane, and its detachment reinitiates the embryological cascades of limb skeletal tissue formation.

Children's periosteum is more developed and thicker than that of adults [30].

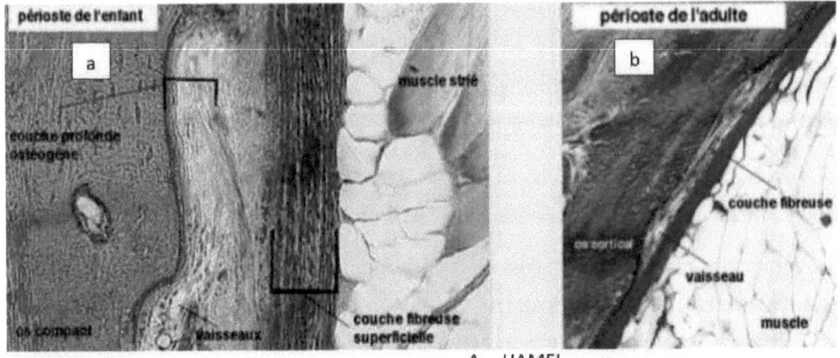

Figure N°11 : Histological aspect of the periosteum (A. Hamel) a- Periosteum in children b- Periosteum in adults

III.2.   Bone Consolidation, Current Data :

In 1987, TEOT set out the basics of bone consolidation in childhood fractures. He showed that, in addition to respect for the fracture hematoma, respect for and role of the periosteum and the importance of centromedullary vascularization, there are other parameters that influence this consolidation. The important role of BMPs (Bone Morphogenic Proteins), osteoclastic balance, ischemia, hypoxia and the role of electrical induction phenomena have been introduced [35].

Bone healing does not depend solely on these biological factors. Bone regeneration relies on three other fundamental elements [36]:

- Progenitor cells
- Growth factors (osteoinduction)
- A suitable environment (osteo-conduction)

GIANNOUDIS' [37] mechanical environment is added to these conditions. These four conditions lead to the modern diamond concept (figure N°12):

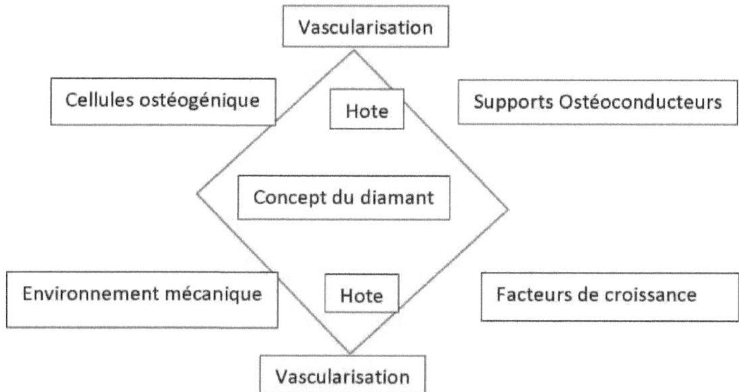

Figure 12: Diamond model integrating the components required for fracture consolidation. Adapted from Giannoudis [37].

Bone consolidation is also conditioned by individual and genetic variations [38] and certain harmful factors such as certain medications, aging and smoking.

Analysis of these components has opened the door to bioengineering developments such as the evolution of internal fixation in the osteosynthesis of long bone fractures and the introduction of stem cell transplantation in osteogenesis imperfecta [39].

This analysis has also led to a biological understanding of the concept of osteosynthesis [40] in:

- Respect for the periosteum
- Respecting the fracture hematoma
- The development of percutaneous surgery
- The elasticity of osteosynthesis devices

These principles are not specific to osteogenesis imperfecta, but are common to all concepts of consolidation.

IV. HISTOLOGY AND PATHOPHYSIOLOGY:

IV.   1. Histology and cytology of normal bone :

Bone tissue is a connective tissue whose composition, organization and dynamics ensure its mechanical support function and its role in mineral homeostasis.

IV.   1.1 Composition of bone tissue :

IV.   1.1.1. The protein framework :

IV.1.1.1.1. Bone collagen:

Collagen fibers account for almost 90% of the total protein matrix of bone. These fibers are made up of micro-fibrils, themselves the result of the alignment of procollagen molecules. The pro-collagen molecule is a heteropolymer arranged in a triple helix: two cx1(I) chains and one $\alpha2(II)$ chain [41], [42].

Type I collagen is the body's most abundant structural protein. It is present in almost all the body's supporting connective tissues (bone, skin, vessels, teeth, ligament, eyes....), which explains the diversity of manifestations in the event of deficiency, as in osteogenesis imperfecta [41], [42].

IV.1.1.1.2. Non-collagenous proteins:

Many non-collagenous proteins present in the bone matrix have been purified and sequenced, but their physiological role is still poorly understood. They account for 10-15% of total bone proteins.

IV.1.1.1.3. Mineral substance:

The inorganic phase of the bone matrix gives bone its rigidity and mechanical strength, and also represents an important mineral reserve. Indeed, around 99% of the body's calcium, 85% of its phosphorus, and between 40 and 60% of its sodium and magnesium are incorporated into the crystals that make up bone mineral substance [41].

In short, bone tissue is characterized by the impregnation of calcium salts on an organic matrix. This matrix is made up of 90% type I collagen fibers. It is the close association between these organic and mineral matrices that gives bone its biomechanical properties. As a result :

- If the mineral phase is removed, the remaining bone retains its shape but loses its rigidity.

- If the organic phase (collagen) is removed, the remaining bone is extremely brittle.

IV. 1.2 Bone Tissue Structures :

IV.1.2.1. Bone texture:

Woven bone is immature, non-lamellar bone characterized by an anarchic arrangement of collagen fibers. It is normally present in embryos and children, where it is gradually replaced by lamellar bone. It is also found in fracture callus, certain primary and secondary bone tumors, osteogenesis imperfecta and Paget's disease. Normal adult bone is made up of lamellar bone resulting from the different orientation of collagen fibers in two contiguous lamellae. This lamellar texture gives bone its mechanical strength[42] :

IV.1.2.2. Bone architecture :

It is organized into compartments [42] :

- Compact bone and trabecular bone differ according to the arrangement of the bone lamellae.
- The endosteum is the intermediate zone between cortical and cancellous bone.
- The periosteum is the outer envelope of the bones.
- a. Os compact :

This is the cortical bone, formed by the juxtaposition of osteons, the elementary structural units of cortical bone, in which the bone lamellae are arranged concentrically around a central canal called Havers' canal, where the vessels circulate. Havers' canals are interconnected by transverse canals known as Volkmann's canals.

- b. Trabecular bone :

Also known as cancellous bone, it consists of a three-dimensional network of bone trabeculae made up of elementary structural units in the form of plates or arches, with a regular lamellar texture. The hematopoietic marrow lies between the bone trabeculae.

IV.1.2.3. Bone cells :

They are responsible for the various phases of bone remodeling [42].

   a.   Osteoclasts :

The osteoclast is the bone cell responsible for resorption. Unlike the osteoblast, it is derived from a hematopoietic precursor.

   b.   Osteoblasts :

At the endosteal surface, the osteoblast is the cell responsible for bone matrix synthesis and apposition, followed by mineralization; in other words, the bone formation process. Its origin is mesenchymal.

   c.   Osteocytes :

They are derived from the transformation of certain osteoblasts embedded in bone tissue. They are essentially involved in the transmission of mechanosensory signals and in exchanges between cells and the microenvironment.

   d.   Border cells :

They cover bone surfaces in the quiescent phase and are involved in communication between the bone surface, the cellular environment and osteocytes embedded in the bone matrix. They also play a role in the initial phase of bone remodeling.

IV. 1.3 Bone shaping and remodeling :

During childhood, bone modelling and remodelling coexist, whereas in adults only remodelling persists.

IV.1.3.1. Bone modelling :

It ensures bone formation in utero and during childhood, until skeletal maturity in adolescence.

It results from two mechanisms: endochondral ossification and membrane ossification.

   a. Endochondral ossification :

It is responsible for the formation of long bones in the embryo. Mesenchymal cells differentiate into chondroblasts and then into chondrocytes, responsible for synthesizing an extracellular matrix rich in proteoglycans and type II collagen, which then calcifies. This calcified cartilage is invaded by vascular buds carrying osteoclast and osteoblast precursor cells. This calcified cartilage is then colonized by osteoblasts, which synthesize immature bone tissue with a woven texture. This immature bone tissue is eventually resorbed by osteoclasts and replaced by lamellar bone tissue [44].

b. Membrane ossification :

Unlike endochondral ossification, mesenchymal cells differentiate directly into osteoblasts, producing a woven bone matrix. Later, following a classic remodeling sequence, this woven bone is progressively replaced by mature lamellar bone [45].

IV.1.3.2. Bone remodelling :

This process preserves the biomechanical properties of bone tissue and ensures mineral homeostasis [26]. The sequence of bone remodeling takes place according to a precise chronology at a single site, resulting from the activity of a basic multicellular unit. This remodeling activity gives rise to the basic units of bone tissue known as osteons in cortical bone and elementary structural units in cancellous bone. It begins with a phase of osteoclast activation, which leads to bone resorption, followed by a transition phase that culminates in the recruitment of osteoprogenitor cells, followed by the formation and mineralization of a new bone matrix. At any given time, around 5% of intracortical surfaces and 20% of trabecular surfaces are undergoing remodeling. This process involves a close coupling between the resorption and formation phases. The average duration of a remodeling sequence is 4 to 6 months.

More recently [46], the living aspect of bone tissue has been explored through the study of the resorption phase of bone remodelling. It was shown that bone cells resorbing the bone matrix did not act randomly, but targeted areas with the weakest mechanical and mineral properties. This behavior, first studied in healthy adult bone tissue, was also observed in the bones of patients suffering from osteogenesis imperfecta. Pathology did not qualitatively modify this behaviour [46].

V. ANATOMOPATHOLOGY:

V. 1. Anatomopathology of bone in osteogenesis imperfecta :

V.   1.1 Macroscopy :

Studies by BULLOGH [47], carried out on autopsies of young children, show that the bones are fragile and friable, and that the epiphyses appear clearly enlarged in relation to the rest of the bone. The secondary ossification centers are deformed, containing small cartilaginous nodules 1 to 4 mm in diameter, and the articular surfaces are irregular.

Conjugation cartilages may be normal, or present abnormalities erasing all or part of their contour. These defects in the CC could explain the severe growth disturbances seen in some patients with osteogenesis imperfecta (Figure N°13).

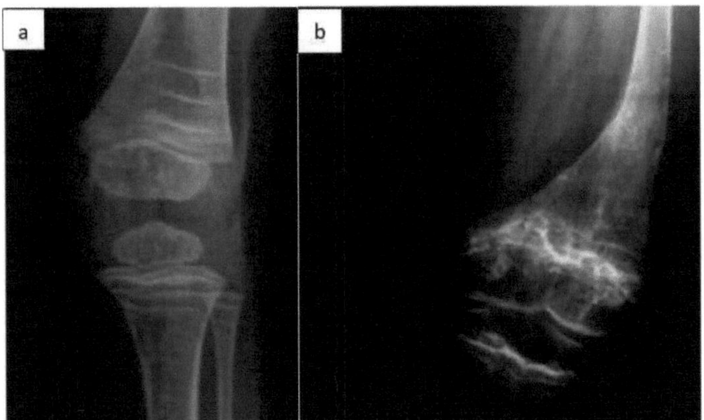

Figure 13: *Radiological appearance of growth plate in osteogenesis imperfecta [personal collection].*
a- Normal growth plate
b- Pathological growth plate (popcorn appearance)

A cross-section of the diaphysis shows :

• A modified periosteum, sometimes thickened but sometimes normal (Figure N°14).

• A very thin cortical layer, which may be missing in some places (figure N°14).

- An enlarged or sometimes obstructed medullary canal.
- A highly vascularized cancellous bone.

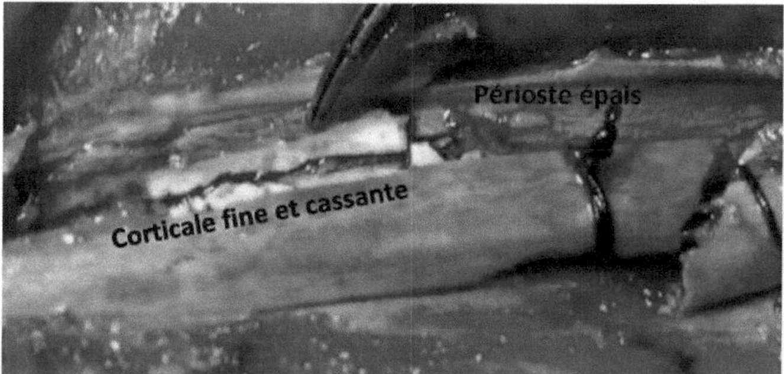

Figure 14: *Intraoperative view of a de-periosteal diaphysis [personal collection].*

V. 1.2 Microscopy:

In children with osteogenesis imperfecta, bone thickness is reduced due to slower bone formation. Bone trabeculae are fewer and abnormally thin [48].

For many authors, osteogenesis imperfecta is a disease of the osteoblast: bone formation is quantitatively and/or qualitatively diminished [49].

As osteoblasts produce less bone structure, the overall rate of bone formation in the trabecular compartment is amplified, due to the increased number of osteoblasts. However, this does not result in a net gain in trabecular bone mass, as bone resorption activity is also increased [50].

Some histological aspects (Figures 15, 16 and 17) are illustrated on samples taken from our patients. This study was carried out in collaboration with the team of anatomopathologists at CHU DOUERA [51].

- un motif lamellaire prédominant fin, avec des zones d'os tissé associé à des fractures.
- les ostéoblastes semblent plus petits, plus sphériques(flèche noire) .
- Les ostéocytes, ovales à arrondis, bien que plus matures en apparence que chez les patients sévèrement atteints, sont plus nombreux, plus grands et moins uniformément répartis dans les trabécules que les ostéocytes chez des témoins (flèches bleu).

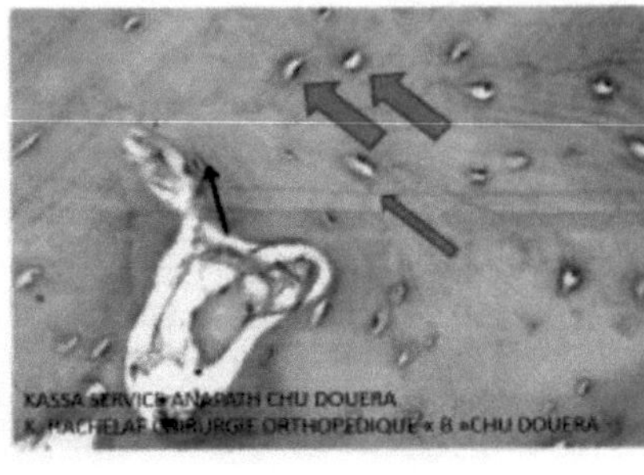

Figure N°15: Histological aspect of a bone sample [personal collection].

- les ostéoblastes tapissant les travées osseuses ont tendance à être moins charnus et fusocellulaire (flèche).
- Les ostéoclastes sont assez rares.
- Cartilage hyperplasique
- Notez les ostéocytes bondés, ovales à arrondis (cercle)

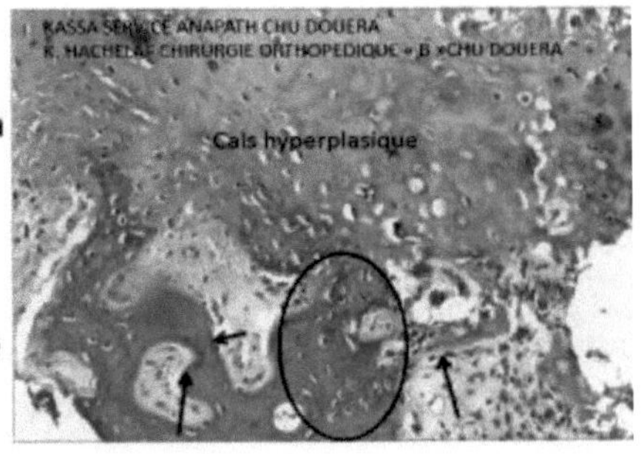

Figure N°16: Histological appearance of a hypertrophic callus in osteogenesis imperfecta [personal collection].

- Le périoste est normalement présent et la couche interne peut être plus importante que la normale
- les ostéoblastes tapissant les travées osseuses ont tendance à être moins charnus et fusocellulaire (flèche).
- Les ostéoclastes sont assez rares.

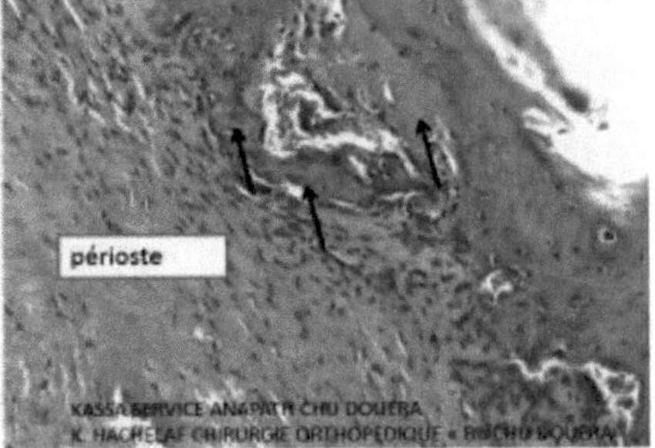

Figure 17: Histological aspect of the periosteum [personal collection].

24

It follows from this study that this is an anomaly in bone formation.

In terms of quality :

- Osteoblasts are more spherical and smaller. They are less fleshy and fusocellular, especially in the bone clast and periosteum.
- Osteocytes are oval, rounded and larger than in normal subjects.
- The periosteum has a more extensive inner layer than in normal subjects.

Quantitative :

- The number of osteoblasts is increased but may produce bone structure.
- Osteocytes are more mature but poorly distributed in the bone trabeculae.
- Osteoclasts are rare, especially in the callus and periosteum.

The combination of these different alterations determines the clinical expression of the disease.

V. 2. Anatomopathology of other tissues

II.   2.1. Eye:

The blue coloration of the sclera is secondary to a reduction in its thickness. The thickness of the cornea is reduced by 25% and that of the sclera by 50%, associated with a defect in the eye's collagen fibers. These fibers have lost their regular striations and present an anarchic organization. As a result, the sclera reveals underlying vessels and choroidal pigments, giving it a bluish appearance [52], [53], [54].

V.2.2. Ear:

The anatomical lesions highlighted in conductive hearing loss in osteogenesis imperfecta were :

- A thickened, enlarged stapes palate fixed in the oval window.
- Dysfunction of the ossicles due to micro-fractures or replacement by fibrous tissue.
- Joint hypermobility of the ossicular chain due to ligament hyperlaxity.
- A thin, flaccid, translucent, sometimes bluish tympanic membrane.

The causes of sensorineural hearing loss are less well known [55].

V.2.3. Dental anomalies :

Dentin is characterized by an irregular, heterogeneous structure, with fine canaliculi running through it. Tubules appear in disordered tufts (Figure N°18). Odontoblasts are usually devoid of ontoblastic extensions, or the latter are very thin. The distribution of canaliculi is anarchic [56], [57], [58].

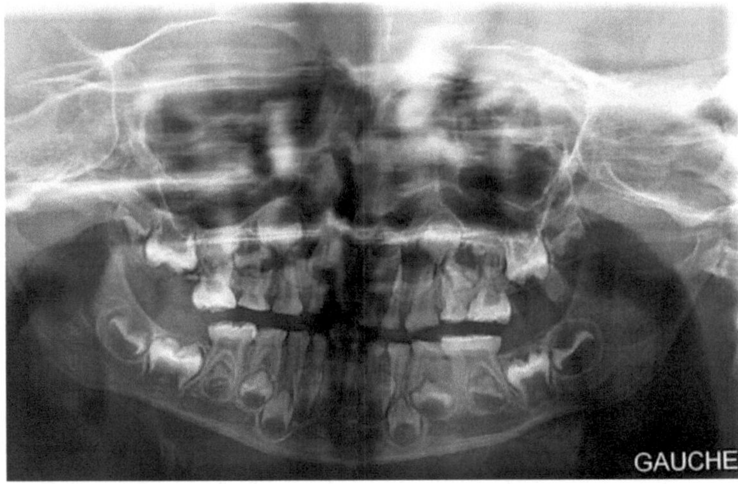

Figure N°18: Radiographic appearance of dentinogenesis imperfecta [personal collection].

VI. GENETICS:

In recent years, genetic and biochemical studies have made numerous advances. These studies have provided new insights into the management of osteogenesis imperfecta. This has given rise to new diagnostic and therapeutic approaches [19], [27], [59].

In around 90% of cases, osteogenesis imperfecta is due to autosomal dominant mutations in the COL1A1, COL1A2 or IFITM5 genes (Figure N°19) [19], [27], [59].

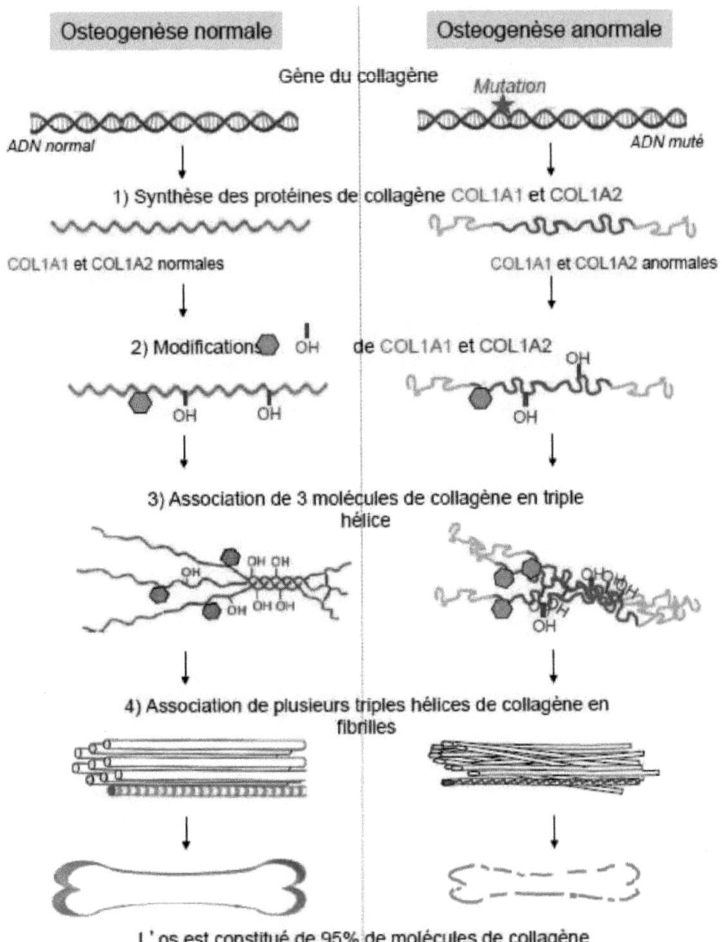

Figure 19: *Comparative diagram of collagen gene mutations [D. Duménil, F. Moreau-Gachelin and M.C. De Vernejoul].*

The remaining *10%* of osteogenesis imperfecta are linked to mutations in autosomal recessive genes.

In the vast majority of osteogenesis imperfecta, bone fragility is evident from childhood, with variable involvement of extra-skeletal connective tissues.

Diagnosis is essentially clinical (capillary fragility, joint hyperlaxity, bluish or greyish sclerae, progressive loss of hearing, cardiac valve damage, etc.) [27], [50].

The majority of these patients have an autosomal dominant mutation in one of the two genes coding for type I collagen, the main collagen in the bone matrix, irrespective of the severity of the phenotype (types I to IV of the SILLENCE classification) [59], [60].

The type I collagen gene is made up of two alpha1 and alpha2 chains associated in a triple helix thanks to the repetitive presence of a glycine residue [19].

Patients with osteogenesis imperfecta carry a mutation in one of the genes encoding the Alpha1 (chromosome 17) and Alpha2 (chromosome 7) chains of type I collagen, and the mutation is inherited in an autosomal dominant fashion.

Studies [61], [62] have shown phenotypic variability for the same mutation. In fact, these phenotypic consequences depend on the location of the mutation, the nature of the substituted amino acid and the type of chain involved.

In the last ten years, rare autosomal recessive forms (around 6-8% of all cases of osteogenesis imperfecta) have been identified, mainly responsible for post-transnational changes in procollagen and collagen fiber maturation, as well as in the homeostasis of bone formation and mineralization [23].

As of September 2016, 14 different genes are known [63]: P3H1, CRTAP, PPIB, FKBP10,SERPINH1, SP7, SERPINF1, BMP1, TMEM38B, WNT1, CREB3L1,TAPT1, PLOD2 and SPARC) or X-linked recessive transmission (PLS3 and MBTPS2). These are moderate to severe forms (Table N°01).

Genes	Heredity	Phenotype (Sillence, Ben Amor, Rauch and Glorieux)	Special features
Structural defects or haploinsufficiency of type 1 collagen			
COL1A1	AD	Types I, II, III, IV	Blue/gray/white sclerae
COL1A2	AD	Types I, II, III, IV	Hyperlaxity, deafness Dentinogenesis imperfecta
Prolyl-3-hydroxylase complex			
CRTAP	AR	Types II, III, IV (VII)	-
LEPRE1	AR	Types II, III (VIII)	Founder" mutation in African-Americans
PPIB	AR	Types II, III, IV (IX)	-
Telopeptide lysyl hydroxylase			
PLOD2	AR	Type III	Pterygium, congenital joint contractures (Bruck type 2 syndrome)
Collagen chaperones			
FKBP10	AR	Types III, IV (XI)	Congenital joint contractures (Bruck type 1 syndrome) possible
SERPINH1	AR	Types II, III (X)	Blue sclerae, dentinogenesis imperfecta
Type 1 collagen maturation			
BMP1	AR	(Type XIII)	Increased bone density, blue sclerae
Bone formation and homeostasis, regulation of bone mass			
SERPINF1	AR	Types III, IV (VI)	Normal at birth, progressive evolution, poor response to bisphosphonates, good response to anti-RANKL antibodies
SP7	AR	Type III (XII)	Delayed tooth eruption
LRP5	AR	Types III, IV	Impaired vision (osteoporosis-pseudoglioma syndrome)
WNT1	AR	Types III, IV (XV)	Progressive course, poor response to bisphosphonates
TMEM38B	AR	Type III (XIV)	-
CREB3L1	AR	Types II-III	-
Unknown functions			
IFITM5	AD	Type V	Hypertrophic calluses, sclerotic metaphyseal bands, calcified interosseous membranes
PLS3	X- linke d	Type I	Early osteoporosis in heterozygous females; osteogenesis imperfecta type I in hemizygous males

Molecular studies can only be carried out after a specialized genetic consultation. This consultation includes genetic investigation of related carriers and genetic counselling. The vast majority of osteogenesis imperfecta are inherited autosomal dominantly. They are associated with a 50% risk of transmission in the offspring of an affected patient; on the other hand, the risk of recurrence in unaffected parents with an affected first child is around 5% (germline mosaicism). More rarely, transmission is autosomal recessive; these forms are associated with a 25% recurrence risk for parents who have already had a child with the disease [19], [27], [59] [63].

Exceptional X-linked forms are usually symptomatic in boys, with occasional minor signs in mothers carrying the mutation. In such cases, genetic counseling is reassuring for the male offspring of an affected man. His daughters will be healthy carriers or only mildly symptomatic [19], [27], [59] [63].

The specialized genetic consultation also enables us to support families in their choices, and to discuss prenatal diagnostic methods and pre-implantation diagnostic techniques.

Molecular studies are currently carried out using NGS (Next Generation Sequencing) panels: targeted sequencing of 19 genes and/or Multiplex Polymerase Chain Reaction (PCR) in specialized molecular genetics laboratories. Molecular studies are relatively long, and their sensitivity is not yet perfect (problem of interpretation of variants and false-negatives). Nonetheless, this study is increasingly proposed to families in order to find out their status and the gene involved, and to answer the question of genetic counseling. It is particularly recommended for people with a severe form who are considering prenatal diagnosis, and for people (fetuses and children) with a severe form whose parents wish to have prenatal diagnosis during a future pregnancy [23], [63].

The "genetic dissection" of the genes involved in osteogenesis imperfecta, which is far from complete, has enormously expanded our knowledge of the biology of the skeleton and bone mineralization, and highlighted target molecules or signaling pathways for new drug therapies, as evidenced by early studies of genotype-guided treatments for osteogenesis imperfecta [64].

The results of genetic and biological research are leading to the choice of a therapeutic molecule adapted to the genetic mutation causing the disease, and to the adaptation of a treatment to certain forms that are not sensitive to bisphosphonates (SERPINF1 and FKBP10), where Denosumab reduces the frequency of fractures and improves bone densitometry and mobility in patients [65]. In the future, the therapeutic indication will be guided by the osteogenesis imperfecta genotype.

VII. DIAGNOSIS:

Type I collagen is the most abundant element in the body, found in the bone matrix, skin, tendons, ligaments, muscles and vascular walls. As a result, any qualitative or quantitative disruption of type I collagen will have an impact not only on bone, but also on various extra-skeletal sites, hence the wide variety of clinical manifestations in osteogenesis imperfecta [18], [23].

These essential clinical manifestations of osteogenesis imperfecta can be divided into two parts:

Skeletal manifestations: of varying severity, these include pain, fractures, bone deformities and growth disorders.

Inconsistent extra-skeletal manifestations: bluish or greyish sclera, dentinogenesis imperfecta, ligament hyper-laxity, skin fragility, vascular fragility, cardiovascular disorders, respiratory disorders, neurological disorders, hearing disorders and deafness, metabolic problems.

These clinical manifestations present a great variability of expression, ranging from simple and moderate forms that can go unnoticed, to major lethal perinatal forms. Their expression can start from intra-uterine life to early childhood, evolving into adulthood [66].

VII.   1. Skeletal Manifestations:

They are directly linked to osteoporosis and its consequences (fractures - deformations); radiologically, they are characterized by excessive bone transparency and very thin cortices (figure N°20).

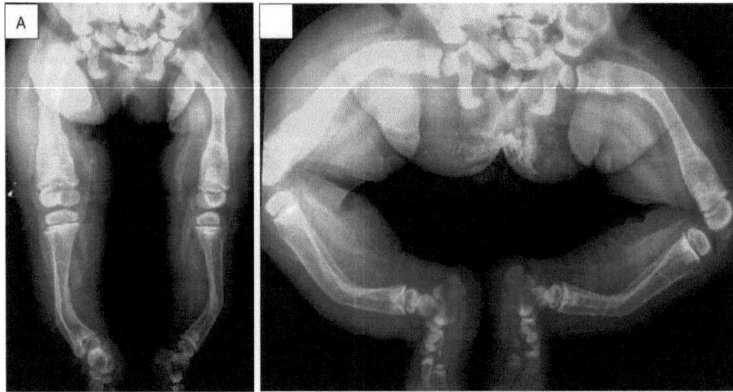

Figure N°20: Radiological image of different bone manifestations in the lower limbs of a 4-year-old child [personal collection].
a- Front X-ray
b- Profile X-ray

Osteoporosis can be quantified by measuring bone density (bone densitometry). These measurements can be made mainly using the DEXA technique [67] and axial densitometry. Quantifying osteoporosis poses problems of measurement. It requires the use of a sensitive device, given the small quantity of bone to be analyzed. Comparison tables are needed, based on the age and, above all, the body surface area of each subject. You need to know the difference between an absolute increase in bone density and a relative increase, which can be seen as a result of bone compression.

VII. 1.1. Pain :

Pain is a frequent symptom of osteogenesis imperfecta. It may be acute, following a fracture. It may be chronic, reflecting the repetition of microfractures or pseudarthrosis on a deformity stock. Vertebral compression or isthmic lysis may be expressed as chronic low back pain [68], [69].

VII. 1.2. Fractures:

Fractures are frequent, constant and of different ages. They vary in severity, from simple cortical fractures to complex commutative fractures, and simple complete fractures with transverse fracture lines and little or no displacement [15], [28].

They can be seen on any bone and occur during intrauterine life, at birth (Fig. N°21), during childhood and into adulthood [66]. They have the particularity of occurring following benign trauma.

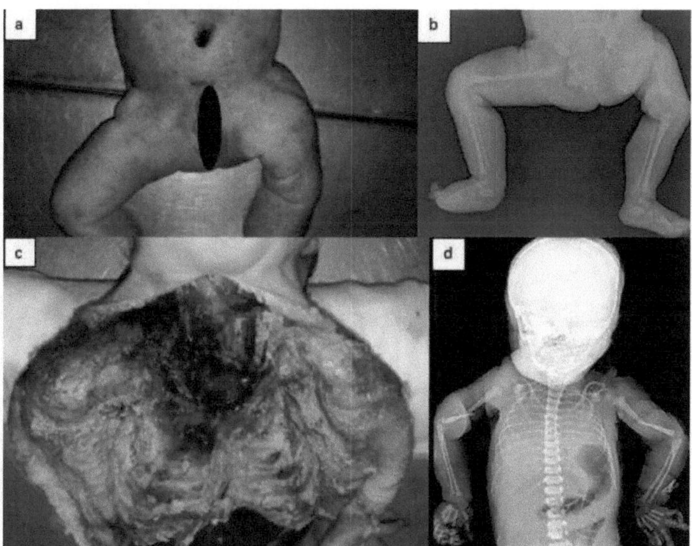

Figure N°21: *Post-mortem autopsy of a child with osteogenesis imperfecta [personal collection].*

a- Deformity of the left thigh b- Fracture of the left femur
c- Rib fractures of different ages

The number of fractures increases around the age of acquisition of walking, stabilizes at puberty and increases again after menopause in adult women [15], [68], [69].

Fracture consolidation in osteogenesis imperfecta is not a problem. It is achieved within the normal timeframe. Consolidation callus is abnormal. Vicious callus consolidation is frequent; the callus may be hypertrophic and often confused with tumoral lesions. It can be a source of deformity. Consolidation may also lead to calcification of the inter-bone membrane [70]. Some authors report a high rate of pseudarthrosis [15], [71].

Avulsion fractures are a special case. They are often seen at the level of the olecranon and anterior tibial tuberosities [15], [72].

VII. 1.3. Deformations :

Bone deformities can be seen all over the skeleton, but most commonly on the long bones. They are either secondary to malunion, or occur spontaneously, due to the inability of these fragile bones to resist muscular traction. As the bone grows, it is unable to stretch the surrounding muscle groups [15], [28], [63], [68].

VII.1.3.1.Limb deformities :

VII.1.3.1.1. Lower limbs :

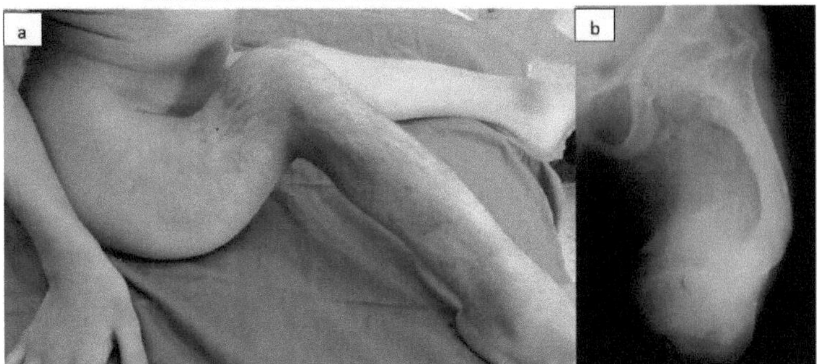

Figure 22: *Lower limb deformity [personal collection].*
a- View of a thigh deformity
b- Front radiograph of a femur deformed in several planes of space

The femur is the most commonly affected bone. Most often, an antero-external crooked deformity develops under the effect of traction from the adductor and hamstring muscles of the thigh (figure N°22).
This curvature is likely to worsen with growth, from a small-radius curvature to a very large one with an extreme radius.
This cruciate deformity is often accompanied by a reorientation of the upper end of the femur into coxa vara. This coxa vara is said to be true when it is secondary to fractures of the base of the neck or the trochanteric region. It is called false coxa vara or induced coxa vara when correction of the femur's diaphyseal deformity corrects the femur's cervicodiaphyseal angle.
At the level of the leg, an anterior or anteromedial crook develops under the effect of the posterior and posterolateral muscles of the leg. This deformity is

known as saber blade deformity. The fibula is often filiform and small [73].

VII.1.3.1.2. Upper limbs

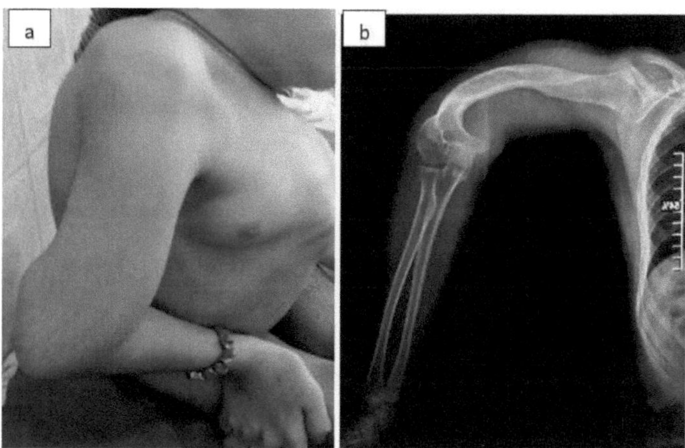

Figure 23: *Upper limb deformity [personal collection].*
a- Side view of a deformed arm
b- Frontal radiology of the two bone segments of the upper limb

These deformities can be seen on the humerus and both forearm bones. They are the result of an imbalance between growth and the inability of the soft, crumbly bone to stretch the surrounding muscles.

In the humerus, these deformities can be oriented in different planes of space (Fig. N°23). Note the anatomical peculiarity of the passage of noble elements, in particular the radial nerve, which runs from back to front in the lower third of the humerus.

The radial nerve may have a variation in position or an unusual pathway within these deformities.

For both forearm bones, in severe forms, gracile, twisted bones with an obstructed medullary canal are often found.

These deformations place the diaphysis in question in a situation of weakness and stress, leading to fractures at the apex of the deformations. The result is a vicious circle of fracture, deformation and fracture.

This vicious circle is a source of deformation, with variable angulation and increasing radius, starting out in one plane of space and becoming multidirectional, sometimes incompatible with the limb's function.

Cases of ulnar pseudarthrosis with radial head dislocation have been reported in the literature [29]. Calcifications of the interosseous membrane may be observed [50].

VII.1.3.1.3. Morphological classifications:

The intertwining of repeated fractures, malunion and deformities of increasing severity will lead to minor or major obstruction of the medullary canal.

MOOREFIELD et al [74] proposed a radiological classification based on the severity of the deformities.

They described three deformation stages of increasing severity:

- Stage I: discreet, with an inclination of less than 20° and virtually normal diaphyseal calibre.
- Stage II: moderate, with inclination between 20° and 60° and moderate diaphyseal thinning.
- Stage III: severe, with inclination greater than 60° and significant diaphyseal taper.

This classification is limited to assessing the size of a deformity and the calibre of the diaphysis, without taking into account associated fractures, the number and orientation of the deformities, the state of the diaphyseal shaft and the impact of these deformities on the upper end of the femur and the coxa vara.

JUSTIN EASOWW and MALA DHARMALINGAM [75] classify bone manifestations into three categories:

- Category I: thin bone and gracile cortex
- Category II: short, thick bone
- Category III: morphological modification of the basin

This classification does not take into account deformities or the quality of the medullary canal.

VII.1.3.1.4 Classification of the orthopaedic surgery department
B, CHU Douera; ALGERIA :

Our radiological analysis is based on the presence or absence of fractures, the angulation of the deformities, the number of curvatures and their orientation in space, the state of permeability of the diaphyseal shaft and the presence or absence of a femoral coxa vara.

Once the results had been collated, we grouped the different bone manifestations into six radiological types of increasing severity (Table N°07):

Type I: Bone without deformity, with or without fracture.

Type II: Bones with simple deformity, angle of curvature less than 30° in a single plane of space, with or without fracture.

Type III: Moderate deformation in two planes of space. Angle of curvature between 30°-50° with or without fracture.

Type IV: Severe deformation in several planes of space, angle of curvature principal > 50°, diaphyseal shaft free, with or without fracture.

TypeV: Severe deformation in several planes of space, angle of curvature principal > 50°, partially obstructed shaft not exceeding one third, with or without fracture

TypeVI: Severe deformation in several planes of space, angle of curvature principal> at 50°, diaphyseal shaft completely obstructed, fine sabre-blade diaphysis. Presence or absence of coxa vara, with or without fracture.

This classification was used when presenting our results in the treatment of limb fractures and deformities in osteogenesis imperfecta at SOFCOT 2018 .

In practical terms, the various radiological parameters are important for surgical planning.

VII.1.3.2 Basin deformations:

The mechanical constraints exerted throughout life on bone fragility in the pelvis will be a source of certain complications [76] [77].

Progressive varus curvature of the upper end of the femur (Fig. N°24 - a) is common, and can lead to major coxa vara deformities, often resulting in recurrent cephalic fractures. It may be complicated by pseudarthrosis of the femoral neck [76] [77].

Acetabular protrusion (Fig. N°24 - b) is more specific to osteogenesis imperfecta, and is a complication often seen in severe forms. Acetabular protrusion is progressive and becomes major, leading to contact between the quadrilateral blades. Acetabular protrusion limits hip mobility [76] [77].

Limited hip mobility associated with pelvic asymmetry contributes to difficulties in standing up, and discomfort in sitting and lying down. Adducted hip retraction makes grooming difficult, and can cause sexual difficulties in women.

Some authors [78] [79] have described visceral complications associated with pelvic deformities.

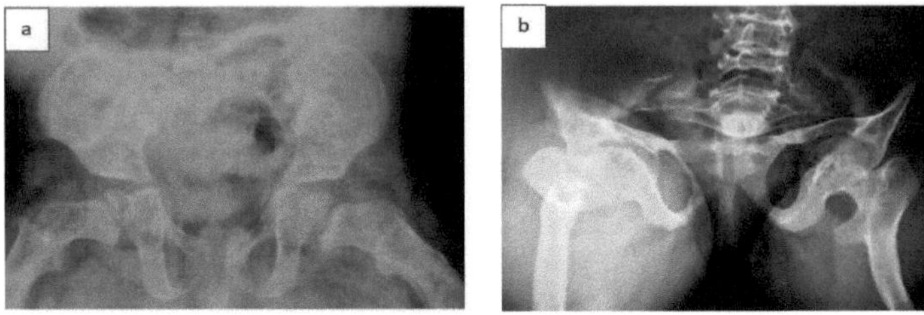

Figure N°24: *X-ray showing pelvic deformities [personal collection] a- X-ray of the pelvis at age 4 b- X-ray of the pelvis at age 16*

VII.1.3.3 Thoracic deformations:

The thorax is frequently deformed, especially in severe forms. The ribs are horizontal, curved and fragile. Lung fields are reduced and airways are deviated (figure N°25).

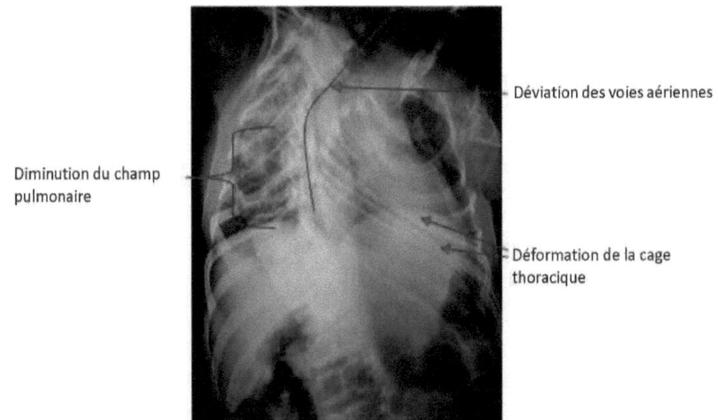

Figure 25: *Chest X-ray illustrating the various thoracic injuries [personal collection].*

Bone calluses of different ages and spinal deformities are present, and the sternum protrudes. The result is a short thorax, with pectus excavatum or carinatum deformities (Figure N°26).

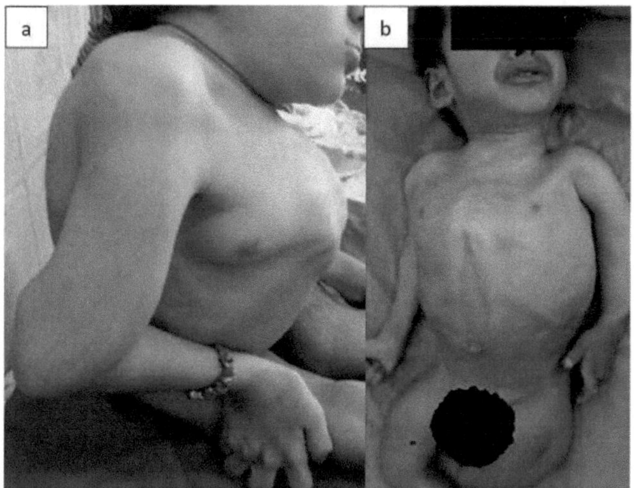

Figure N°26: *Thoracic deformity [personal collection]: a- wishbone deformity in a 16-year-old girl b- wishbone deformity in a 06-year-old boy*

The combination of spinal deformity and thoracic involvement results in a severe reduction in respiratory capacity, leading to respiratory failure. These respiratory disorders are at the root of the difficulties inherent in anesthesia [80].

VII.1.3.4 Spinal deformities:

Spinal deformities in osteogenesis imperfecta are linked to bone fragility, vertebral compression, ligament hyperlaxity and growth failure. The height of the vertebrae is reduced, resulting in platyspondyly [81], [82]. The vertebra may be wedge-shaped or take on the appearance of a biconcave lens. The result is a disturbance of spinal statics in the form of kyphosis, scoliosis or cypho-scoliosis (Figure N°27). Whether scoliosis, kyphosis or cypho-scoliosis is combined with thoracic deformities, respiratory capacity is impaired, with a reduction in vital capacity.

The severity of spinal deformities depends on several factors:

- The severity of osteogenesis imperfecta.
- Thoracic deformities.
- Patient's age.
- Degree of vertebral collapse.
- Bone densitometry
- Ligament hyper laxity.

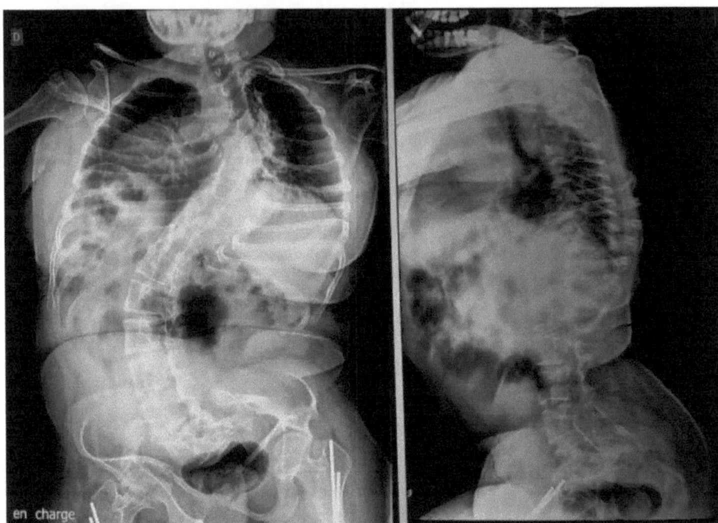

Figure 27: Spinal deformities: Cyphoscoliosis [personal collection].

VII.1.3.5 Skull deformations:

Macrocephaly is common, with transverse enlargement of the skull (a broad, domed forehead). It combines a broad, rounded forehead with a small chin, giving patients a triangular face [15] [18].

Radiologically (Fig. 28), the skull shows numerous Wolmian bones corresponding to a mosaic of primary ossification islands within the membranous bone. The occiput may be flattened.

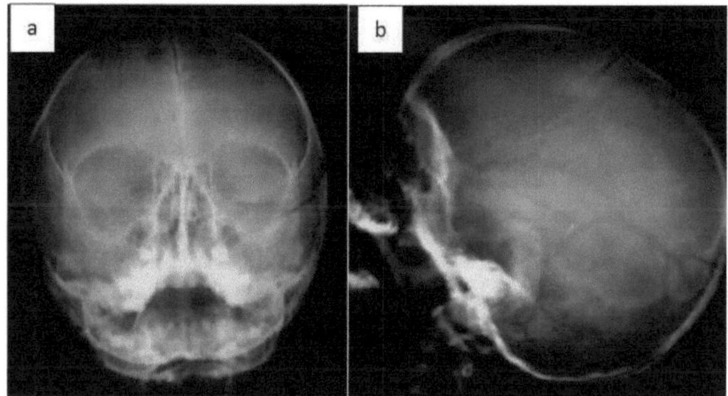

Figure 28: Skull morphology [personal collection]: a- Front skull b- Side skull

Basilar impression (Fig. N°29) is a deformity that combines an upward displacement of the foramen magnum with the first vertebrae appearing to be sunken into the cranial cavity. It is a worrying deformity, often seen in adolescence, causing headaches, sharp reflexes and weakness of the lower limbs [15] [18].

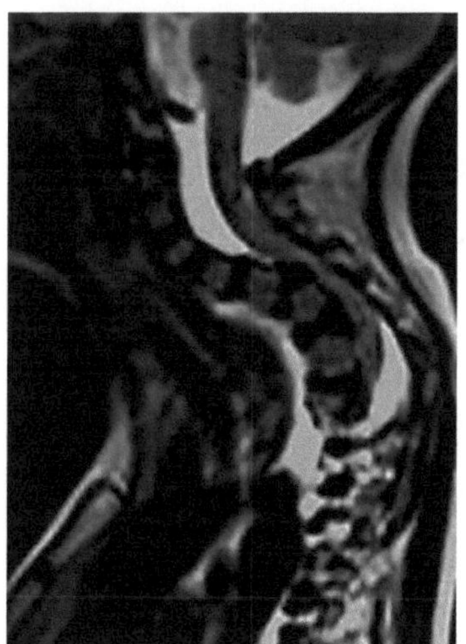

Figure N°29: MRI image of a basilar impression [collection G. FINIDORI].

VII.1.3.6 Small size:

Height deficiency is common in osteogenesis imperfecta (Figure N°30), and its severity depends on the type of osteogenesis imperfecta: it is normal or slightly reduced in type I. It can be very severe in type III.
Statural insufficiency may be absent or severe [15], [18], [28].

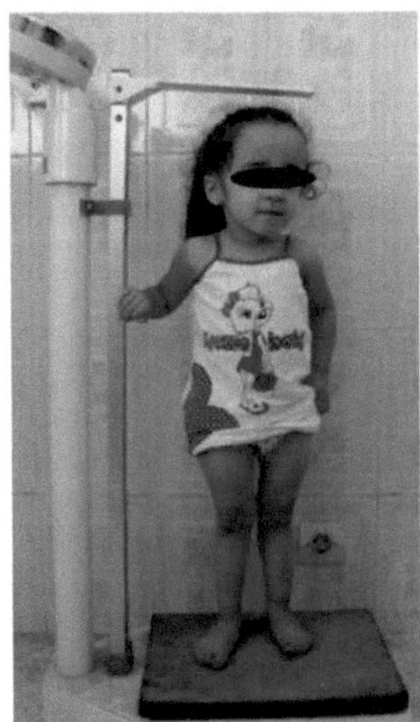

Figure N°30: representative image of a girl of small stature [personal collection].

VII.2 Extra-skeletal manifestations :

They have been reported by numerous authors [15], [28], [83].

VII.2.1. Sclerotic blues:

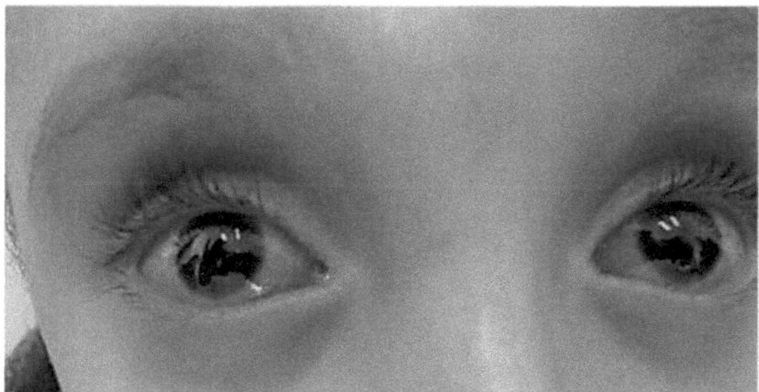

Figure N°31: *image of blue sclera [personal collection].*

Bluish discoloration of the sclera (Figure N°31) is secondary to excessive transparency of the sclera. This discoloration is variable in intensity and evolves over the years.

EDDOWERS was the first to report the relationship between blue sclera and osteogenesis imperfecta. The appearance of sclera can be normal or physiological in newborns. This clinical manifestation is neither specific to osteogenesis imperfecta, nor to type I collagen anomalies [52], [53].

Hyperopia is common [15].

Myopia is not associated with osteogenesis imperfecta [18].

VII.2.2. Dentinogenesis imperfecta :

Dentinogenesis is disrupted (dentinogenesis imperfecta), but the manifestation depends on the type of osteogenesis imperfecta.

It is best seen in deciduous teeth. These are brittle, amber, grey or yellow-brown teeth (Fig. N°32), bulging in a tulip or bell shape [84], and radiology shows obliterated pulp canals [85]. Enamel and dentine are fragile, and teeth wear rapidly. Oral hygiene and the use of fluoride remain the preventive measures of choice. Treatment should be carried out by a dentist specializing in dentinogenesis.

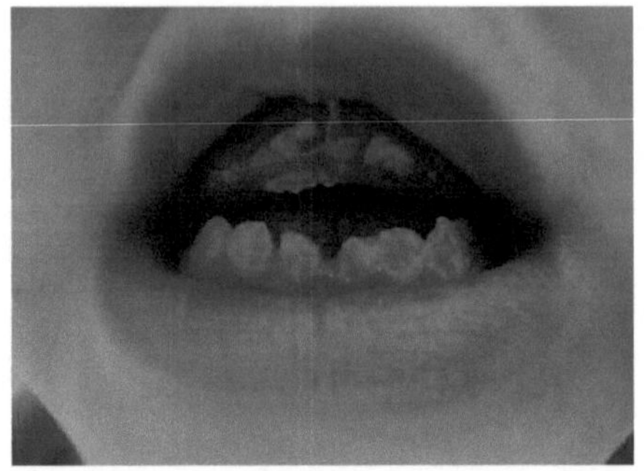

Figure N°32: Dentinogenesis imperfecta [personal collection].

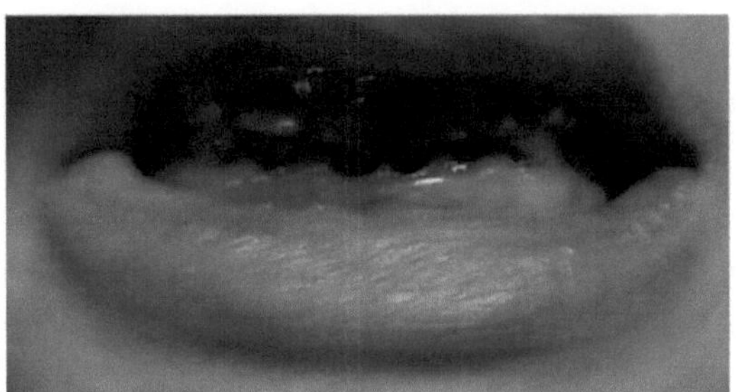

VII.2.3. Ligament laxity and hyperlaxity:

Hyperlaxity is virtually constant in osteogenesis imperfecta, and poses no clinical problems. Occasionally, hyperlaxity can compromise joint stability (flatfoot, recurvatum of the knees...) and cause easy sprains.
It can affect standing and walking. Hyperlaxity is an aggravating factor in spinal statics disorders.
This hyperlaxity may be cutaneous or musculo-ligamentary (Figure N°33).
When ligament laxity is absent or replaced by joint contracture associated with osteoporosis, BRUCK syndrome should be considered [86] [87].

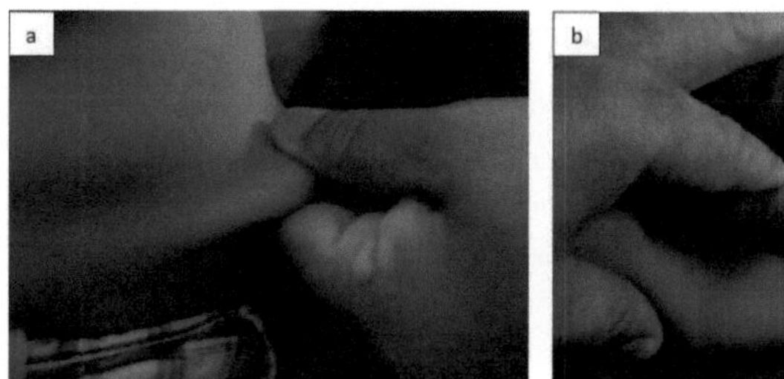

Figure 33: Clinical signs of hyperlaxity [personal collection] a- Cutaneous hyperlaxity b-Hyperflexion of the thumb

VII.2.4. Metabolic abnormalities:

These abnormalities have been known for a long time [88]. They are linked to increased basal metabolism, resulting in heat intolerance, elevated basal temperature, excessive sweating (hypersudation), tachycardia and tachypnea. These symptoms may give rise to fears of malignant hyperthermia. The pathogenesis of these disorders remains unknown.
Spontaneously resolving hypermetabolic reactions may be seen during general anesthesia, but with no increased risk of malignant hyperthermia according to some authors [89].

VII.2.5. Cardiovascular abnormalities :

Cardiovascular manifestations are rare. They are expressed later and less clearly than in hereditary connective tissue disorders such as Marfan syndrome and Ehrlers Danlos syndrome. Type I collagen deficiency can lead to valvular and aortic lesions [90]. This deficiency can be the cause of rupture of the heart chamber, aorta and cerebral blood vessels [91].

Bruises, hematomas and epistaxis are common in children with osteogenesis imperfecta. Cerebral haemorrhages have been reported in the literature. These disorders are associated with fragile capillary walls and impaired platelet function.
These cardio-circulatory abnormalities are more frequent in adulthood, which is why it is advisable to perform systematic ultrasound examinations in patients with osteogenesis imperfecta entering adulthood at around 10 years of age, and to explore platelet function preoperatively [92].

VII.2.6. Respiratory abnormalities:

Bronchopulmonary infection, inhalation pneumonitis, acute respiratory failure and chronic respiratory failure are all complications that can be seen in children with osteogenesis imperfecta. Respiratory failure is a frequent cause of death in osteogenesis imperfecta [93].

These respiratory complications are secondary:
- Bone deformations in the ribcage (figure N°34-1), which create an imbalance between respiratory mechanics and muscular movements.
- Compression of the airways by various spinal and costo-sternal deformations (figure N° 34-2).
- Neurological disorders caused by bulbar compression, common in severe osteogenesis imperfecta in adolescence [94].

In severe cases, a restrictive syndrome may develop as a result of reduced lung fields secondary to severe thoraco-spinal deformities. Respiratory capacity is reduced, and collapsed lung fields are sometimes incompatible with life (figure N°34-3) [95].

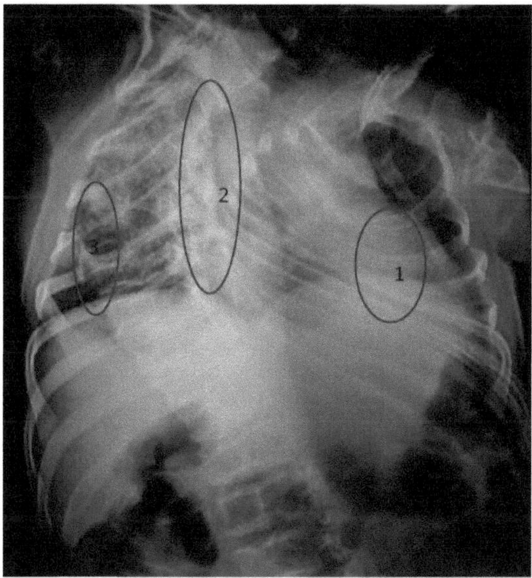
Figure 34: *costo-sternal deformities [personal collection].*
1. *Rib deformities*
2. *Sternal deformity*
3. *Collapsed lung field*

VII.2.7. Hearing anomalies :

Deafness is seen in 22 to 58% of patients with osteogenesis imperfecta, 20% of whom are unaware of their condition. It appears progressively. It is most often bilateral and late in onset. Its onset varies between the ages of 15 and 40. The deafness may be conductive due to damage to the stapes, sensorineural or mixed [63], [94].

Some authors [96] recommend systematic screening at the age of 10 and then every three years, while others recommend screening for suspected deficiency.

Treatment may require a hearing aid or surgery with a cochlear implant [97]. Hearing loss due to serous otitis in infants with osteogenesis imperfecta appears to be more common than in the general population [63].

VII.2.8. Skin abnormalities:

The skin is thin, transparent and translucent. It is the frequent site of rapidly spreading hematoma secondary to minimal trauma. Healing is atrophic. The scar tends to widen, taking on an atypical "cigarette-paper" appearance [98].

VII.2.9. Neurological abnormalities.

Certain nerves can be compressed by bony deformities, such as the basilar impression. This can lead to recurrent headaches and hyper-reflexia in adolescents. This situation requires regular MRI monitoring, sometimes even leading to spinal cord release and occipito-cervical fixation [99].
Hydrocephalus with ventricular dilatation occurs in 20-30% of cases. It is often asymptomatic. In rare symptomatic forms, cerebrospinal fluid diversion is exceptionally necessary [99].
Some authors [100] report cortical atrophy, syringomyelia and rare cases of epilepsy.
In newborns, there may be a risk of sub dural or extra dural hematoma at birth.

VII.2.10. Renal microlithiasis :

Hypercalciuria is usually associated with hyperremodeling of bone. Renal micro-lithiasis is generated by this hypercalciuria. Renal ultrasonography is recommended as part of the initial work-up of a child with osteogenesis imperfecta.
[101] .

VII.2.11. Psycho-social problems :

Children with osteogenesis imperfecta and their families are subject to constraints in terms of education, care and social life. These children grow up in a particular context, fraught with painful episodes (fracture, hospitalization, surgery and delayed schooling). These children suffer from society's view of their disabilities.
[102] .
The development of deformities in adolescence disrupts body image, making it difficult for many children and their families to accept.
Children should regain their self-confidence as quickly as possible and quickly

return to their school environment, play areas and normal life [102].
On the other hand, parents have to cope with the diagnosis of the disease and learn to live with it.

They have to deal with all the constraints this entails:
- Professional absenteeism to accompany their child.
- The cumbersome nature of the treatment (pediatrician, rehabilitator and surgeon), making it necessary to concentrate appointments in a single multidisciplinary consultation.

Support for osteogenesis imperfecta families starts with good dissemination of information and communication between the various parties involved [102].

VII.3 Clinical classifications :

Osteogenesis imperfecta is a pathology with variable and non-specific manifestations. Several authors have taken an interest in it:

VII.3.1. LOOSER classification :

LOOSER [103] in 1906 described two forms of osteogenesis imperfecta depending on the age at which the first fractures occurred:
- osteogenesis imperfecta congenita or PORAK and DURANTE disease, fractures can be seen at birth.
- osteogenesis imperfecta tarda or LOBSTEIN disease, fractures are seen after the perinatal period.

VII.3.2. MAROTEAU classification :

Pierre MAROTEAU [104] also distinguishes between two forms: those with an ante-natal onset and those detected after birth.

Ante-natal onset: These are children who, from birth, have fractures or deformities of the long bones, or even the spine and skull. These deformities suggest bone fragility in utero.
MAROTEAU and his team [104] distinguish three forms:
- The lethal form.
- The severe form.
- The regressive form.

Forms discovered after birth: These are divided into three groups:
- The most complete generalized forms.
- Elective forms.
- Moderate forms.

VII.3.3. SILLENCE classification modified by GLORIEUX :

The evolution of clinical, genetic, biochemical and histological studies has shown a diversity of manifestations of this heterogeneous pathology.

The SILLENCE classification is the first to define 4 types of osteogenesis imperfecta. It is based on the clinical manifestations and mode of transmission of the disease [52]. GLORIEUX introduced three further groups of patients with distinct genetic and histological clinical features. Currently, 7 types of osteogenesis imperfecta are defined (Table N°02) [50], [70].

Classification de l'ostéogenèse imparfaite (OI) de Sillence et de Glorieux.	
OI de type I (bénigne)	• Fractures par suite de traumatismes minimes • Sclérotique bleutée • Malformation minime des os longs • Taille normale ou quasi-normale • Possibilité de dentinogenèse imparfaite
OI de type II (mortelle)	• Fractures intra-utérines • Chapelet costal • Sclérotique bleutée • Fémur large et court • Détresse respiratoire • Décès pendant la période périnatale
OI de type III (grave)	• Fractures fréquentes par suite de traumatismes minimes • Sclérotique de couleur variable • Taille extrêmement petite • Grave malformation des membres • Scoliose • Faciès triangulaire • Dentinogenèse imparfaite fréquente
OI de type IV (modérée)	• Fractures par suite de traumatismes minimes • Sclérotique de couleur variable • Taille modérément petite • Malformation modérée des membres • Scoliose • Possibilité de dentinogenèse imparfaite
OI de type V	• Fractures par suite de traumatismes minimes • Sclérotique normale • Calcification de la membrane interosseuse de l'avant-bras ou de la jambe • Bande métaphysaire dense sous la plaque de croissance • Callogenèse hypertrophique par suite de fractures ou de bâtonnets • Intramédullaires • Absence de dentinogenèse imparfaite
OI de type VI	• Fractures par suite de traumatismes bénins • Sclérotique normale • Élévation modérée du taux de phosphatase alcaline • Stries de Looser (pseudofractures) visibles à la radiographie • Absence de dentinogenèse imparfaite • Absence d'os wormiens Plus • Absence de rachitisme
OI de type VII	• Fractures par suite de traumatismes bénins • Sclérotique normale • Absence de dentinogenèse imparfaite • Coxa vara • Rhizomélie (brièveté des racines des membres supérieurs et inférieurs)

***Table N°02:** SILLENCE and GLORIEUX classification [52], [70].*

VII.3.4. SILLENCE classification modified by RAUCH and GLORIEUX :

Modern studies have made it possible to relate the numerous genetic mutations, whether quantitative or qualitative, and to take into account dominant mutations as well as the numerous genetic defects and their phenotypes [50], [105], (Table N°03).

Type	Clinical severity	Typical features	Typically associated mutations	Relative incidence*
I	Mild non-deforming OI	Normal height or mild short stature; blue sclera; no DI	Premature stop codon in COL1A1	47%
II	Perinatal lethal	Multiple rib and long-bone fractures at birth; marked deformities; broad long bones; low density of skull bones on x-rays; dark sclera	Glycine substitutions in COL1A1 or COL1A2	–
III	Severely deforming	Very short; triangular face; severe scoliosis; grayish sclera; DI	Glycine substitutions in COL1A1 or COL1A2	18%
IV	Moderately deforming	Moderately short; mild to moderate scoliosis; grayish or white sclera; DI	Glycine substitutions in COL1A1 or COL1A2	27%
V	Moderately deforming	Mild to moderate short stature; dislocation of radial head; mineralized interosseous membrane; hyperplastic callus; white sclera; no DI	unknown	4%
VI	Moderately to severely deforming	Moderately short; scoliosis; accumulation of osteoid in bone tissue, fish scale pattern of bone lamellation; white sclera; no DI	unknown	3%
VII	Moderately deforming to perinatal lethal	Severity ranging from death in first days of life to mild short stature. Short humeri and femora; white sclera; no DI	CRTAP	1%

Table N°03: Sillence classification modified by Rauch and Glorieux [50].

VII.4. Positive diagnosis:

The diagnosis of osteogenesis imperfecta is based on a combination of clinical, radiological and biological factors [28], [63], [94] :

VII.4.1. Antenatal diagnosis

Antenatal diagnosis of osteogenesis imperfecta [66], [106] is often made using ultrasound (Figure N°35), sometimes aided by radiography of uterine contents and new molecular biology techniques [107], [108], [109].

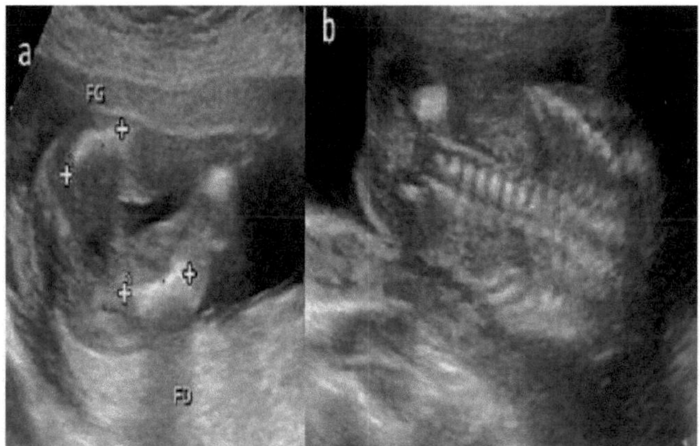

Figure 35: Antenatal ultrasound at 17 weeks of amenorrhea [109] a- Short curved femur
b- Flattened appearance of vertebral bodies

The various ultrasonographic signs of osteogenesis imperfecta are summarized in
Table N°04.

Intrauterine growth retardation
Hydramnios
Cephalic anomalies :
- Hydrocephalus.
- Macrocephaly.
- Spontaneous cephalic deformation or deformation caused by ultrasound probe pressure.
- Thinning and low echogenicity of the bony vault.
- Maximum cephalic deflection.
Thoracic abnormalities :
- Thorax small and narrow.
- Reduced acoustic shadowing of coastlines.
- Fracture and bone callus.
Limb anomalies :
- Dwarfism: obvious and early in type L, not very marked in types R and S.
- Fractures and bone calluses.
- Marked limb deformity.
- Reduced acoustic shadowing of long bones.

Table N°04: Ultrasonographic signs of osteogenesis imperfecta [109].

X-rays of the uterine contents (figure N°36) confirm the poor mineralization of the long bones and skull, with no visualization of the fetal skeleton at all, fractures, bone calluses, deformations and the bamboo-like appearance of the ribs. Interpretation of the images remains difficult and must be performed by an expert.

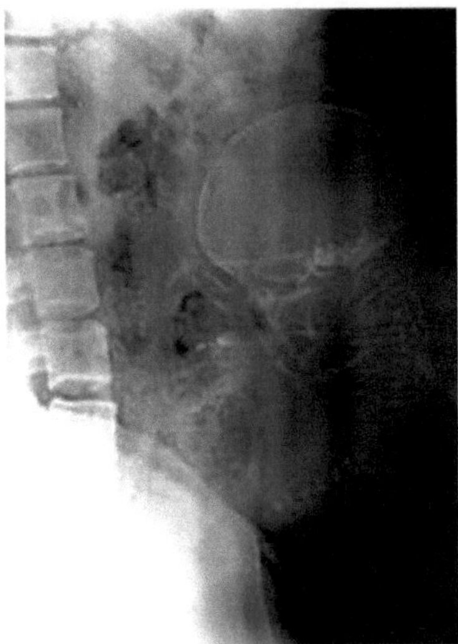

Figure N°36: Radiograph of uterine contents at 38 weeks' gestation (fetus with osteogenesis imperfecta) [108].

Trophoblastic biopsy is an examination carried out between "11 and 14" weeks of amenorrhea. It enables a diagnosis of osteogenesis imperfecta to be made: either by biochemical analysis of type I collagen, synthesized by chorionic villus fibroblasts, or by analysis of fetal DNA by molecular biology [110].

VII.4.2. Post-natal diagnosis

VII.4.2.1 Clinical arguments:

The clinical examination must be complete, combining a police history investigating the evolutionary characteristics of the fractures and their mechanisms, with a full morphological examination (figure N°37).

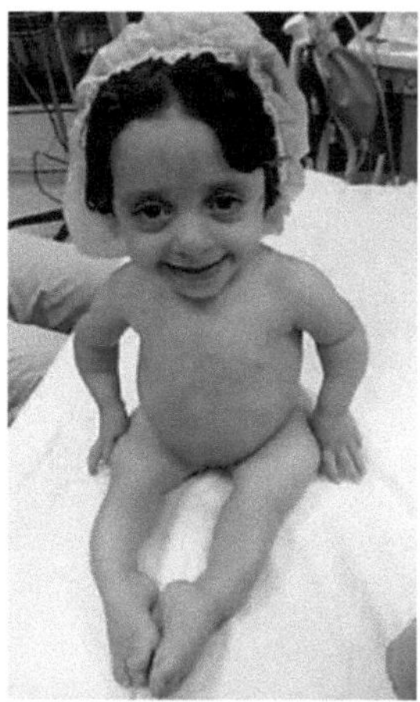

Figure N°37: *Morphological appearance of osteogenesis imperfecta. [Personal collection]*

The diagnosis is clinical [28], [63], [94], and is strongly suggested by the association of :

> ➢ Easy, frequent, repeated, multiple fractures of different ages following minor trauma (Figure N°38).

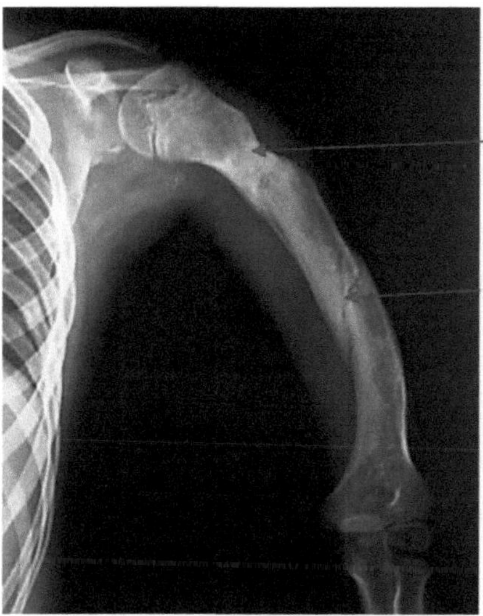

> Minor, inconsistent signs that vary from patient to patient:

- Bluish sclera: this is a non-specific sign. Its absence does not rule out osteogenesis imperfecta.

- Dentinogenesis imperfecta is common. X-rays of the pulp canals can help in the diagnosis.

- Deformities (curvature of long bones, thoracic protrusion, kyphoscoliosis).

- Progressive statural shift.

- Transparent, fragile skin, easy to bruise.

- Vascular fragility.

- Hyperlaxity and multiple sprains.

- Hearing loss (exceptional in children, present in around 50% of adults).

These arguments are reinforced by the presence of the same symptoms in a first-degree relative (parents, siblings).

VII.4.2.2 Radiological and densitometric arguments :

The radiological work-up should include, as a minimum, front and side x-rays of the skull, long bones, dorsolumbar spine and costal grid. The radiograph should focus on the most significant deformity (figure N°39).

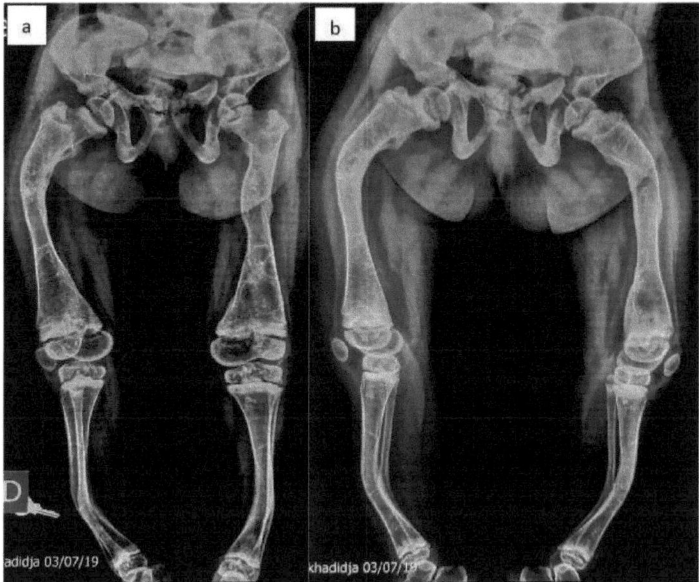

Figure 39: X-ray showing bone deformities in the lower limbs [personal collection] a- Front view b- Profile view

Other radiographs may be clinically guided.

The radiological workup will look for :

- Gracile, osteoporotic bone, thin, transparent cortex.
- Fresh diaphyseal fracture or fracture of different ages, fracture sequelae, sometimes periosteal apposition on long bones, but also metaphyseal tearing (olecranon - anterior tibial tuberosity).
- Platyspondyly, vertebral compression and kyphoscoliosis
- Diaphyseal curvatures and deformities. The number and extent of curvatures must be assessed.
- The state of the diaphyseal shaft, which may be free or partially or totally obstructed.

- Presence or absence of hypertrophic callus, signs of delayed consolidation and presence or absence of pseudarthrosis
- A deformed pelvis with femoral coxa vara with or without acetabular protrusion.

- Deformities of the ribs and sternum; in severe forms, a major wishbone-shaped thoracic deformity.
- A short, transversely enlarged skull and Wormian bones.
- Popcorn calcifications (Fig. N°40): these are intraosseous calcifications resulting from microtraumatic fragmentation and disordered maturation of the growth plate. They occur in the metaphyseal and epiphyseal regions close to the knee (lower end of the femur and upper end of the tibia). They may contribute to femoral growth deficiency and leg length discrepancy [111], [112].

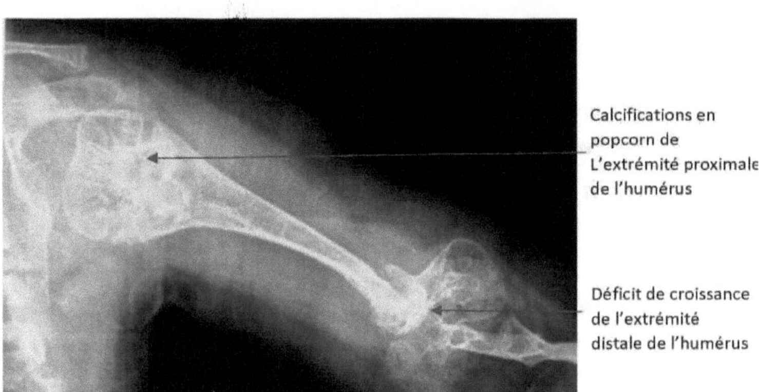

Figure N°40: *Popcorn calcification of humeral growth plate [personal collection].*

- Dense metaphyseal bands: these are hyperdense striae located in metaphyseal zones. They are present in children treated for osteogenesis imperfecta with bisphosphonates and in type V osteogenesis imperfecta regardless of treatment (Figure N°41).

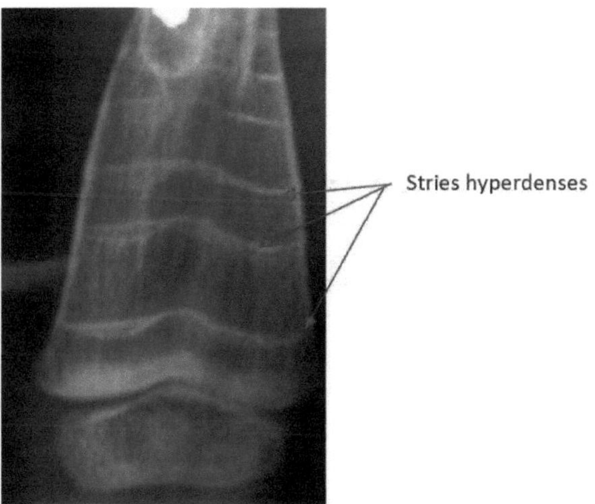

Figure N°41: *Dense metaphyseal bands [personal collection].*

- Hypertrophic callus and calcification of the interosseous membrane (figure N°42).

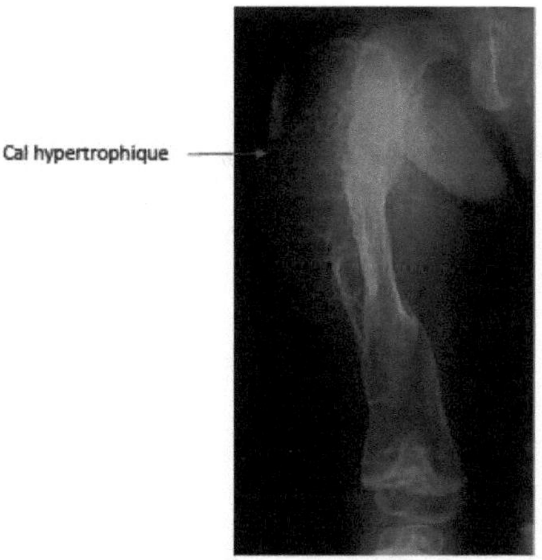

Figure N°42: *X-ray of femur with hypertrophic callus [Personal collection].*

Radiological assessment can be difficult, given the extent of the deformities and the risk of fractures in fragile bones.

Bone densitometry:

Bone densitometry using two-photon X-ray absorptiometry (DEXA) is currently the optimal method for detecting decreased bone mineral density.

BMD can be proposed after 5 years. It shows a decrease in bone mineral density correlated with sex and age. The Z-score is considered in children.

Bone densitometry (BMD) can confirm bone demineralization, but is not necessary for the diagnosis of osteogenesis imperfecta. However, it is an effective means of monitoring medical treatment in osteogenesis imperfecta [15] [18] [63].

VII.4.2.3. Biological arguments :

- **Phosphocalcic balance :**

In most cases, the phosphocalcic profile is normal. This test helps exclude other etiologies of brittle osteopathy, such as hypophosphatasia, metabolic rickets and Paget's disease.

- **Other biological tests:**

The determination of markers of bone resorption and reconstruction in serum can help in the diagnosis of osteogenesis imperfecta [113].

The most frequently dosed bone formation markers are :

- Alkaline phosphatase, osteocalcin, C-terminal (carboxy) propeptide and N-terminal (amino) propeptide of procollagen I.
- The most frequently assayed markers of bone resorption are hydroxyproline and collagen-bridging molecules and their telopeptides (pyridinoline and deoxypyridinoline).

- **Genetics and molecular biochemistry:**

Molecular studies can only be carried out after a specialized genetic consultation. It is indicated during genetic investigation of relatives with osteogenesis imperfecta, and during genetic counselling of parents wishing to procreate. This molecular study is currently carried out by NGS (Next Generation Sequencing) panel: targeted sequencing of 19 genes and/or Multiplex PCR (polymerase chain reaction) in specialized laboratories [23], [63].

These studies are long, costly and not yet perfectly sensitive. There is still a problem of interpretation of variants and false-negatives [23], [63].

Genetic dissection of the genes involved in osteogenesis imperfecta has expanded our knowledge of skeletal biology and bone mineralization. It has opened up new therapeutic avenues, as in the case of certain forms that are not sensitive to bisphosphonates, and as demonstrated by studies on genotype-guided treatment of osteogenesis imperfecta [64].

VII.5. Differential diagnosis :

Osteogenesis imperfecta can be confused with a number of pathologies. This confusion may vary with age.

VII.5.1. During Pregnancy :

In the case of fractures, the diagnosis is much more in favour of osteogenesis imperfecta. However, in the case of curved femurs, the diagnosis of osteogenesis imperfecta must be distinguished from compomelic dysplasia and STUVE-WIDEMANN syndrome. In this case, the presence of skull deformability visible on ultrasound argues in favour of osteogenesis imperfecta [15], [18].

VII.5.2. At birth :

VII.5.2.1 Hyperphosphatasia:

Hyperphosphatasia or "juvenile Paget's disease" is characterized by extremely high bone turnover. Serum alkaline phosphatase levels are very high. Bone fragility is severe, with large diaphyses. Its autosomal recessive inheritance is linked to a mutation in the TNFRSF11B gene [18].

VII.5.2.2 Hypophosphatasia:

The clinical expression of hypophosphatasia is highly variable, ranging from neonatal death (absence of bone demineralization) to pathological fractures in adults, reflecting moderate to severe bone fragility. Serum alkaline phosphatase levels are very low, as is the presence of phosphoethanolamine in urine. Autosomal dominant or recessive transmission is due to a mutation in the ALPL gene.

Osteogenesis imperfecta can also be confused with hyperparathyroidism, mucolipidosis and dysplasia with bone gracility [18].

VII.5.3. In childhood :

VII.5.3.1 SILVERMAN syndrome:

Battered child syndrome is the most common cause of fractures, especially in the first year of life [114].

Differential diagnosis is difficult when familial bone fragility is unknown. There is a risk that the diagnosis of a battered child will be overlooked, or that osteogenesis imperfecta will be misdiagnosed and unjustified legal action taken against innocent parents.

Bone densitometry and type I collagen analysis can sometimes contribute to the diagnosis.

VII.5.3.2 Primary osteoporosis in children:

VII.5.3.2.1. Juvenile idiopathic osteoporosis:

Juvenile idiopathic osteoporosis is a transient, non-hereditary osteoporosis in children, with no extra-skeletal signs. It affects boys and girls between the ages of 7 and 12. Spontaneous recovery occurs after 3 to 5 years. Spinal deformities and severe functional disability may persist [115].

VII.5.3.2.2. Osteoporosis syndrome - pseudo glioma:

It is characterized by low bone mass, frequent fractures, limb deformities, ligament hyperlaxity and short stature.

Eye involvement (retinal pseudogliomas, glaucoma and vitreous hyperplasia) is specific to the disease. It causes severe visual impairment. The syndrome is autosomal recessive and is associated with mutations in the LRP5 gene. [116], [117].

VII.5.3.2.3. COLE-CARPENTER syndrome:

It is a disease of unknown transmission and genetic defect, characterized by osteoporosis and severe bone fragility, short stature, hydrocephalus, craniostenosis leading to acrocephaly and exophthalmos [118].

VII.5.3.2.4. Panostotic fibrous dysplasia:

This is the extreme form of polyostotic fibrous dysplasia. It is linked to a somatic mutation in codon 201 of the gene coding for GNAS. The severity of bone fragility, deformity and short stature clinically resemble osteogenesis imperfecta type III.

On radiology, bone lesions are lacunar and the bone framework is irregular. Low blood phosphorus levels, normal in patients with osteogenesis imperfecta, are typical of panostotic dysplasia [15], [18], [51], [56].

VII.5.3.2.5. BRUCK syndrome:

This syndrome associates variable osteoporosis, bone fragility, arthrogryposis and sometimes limb pterygia (figure N°43). Transmission is autosomal recessive. Some cases are linked to a mutation in the gene coding for a protein with lysyl-hydroxylase activity, which is deficient [119].

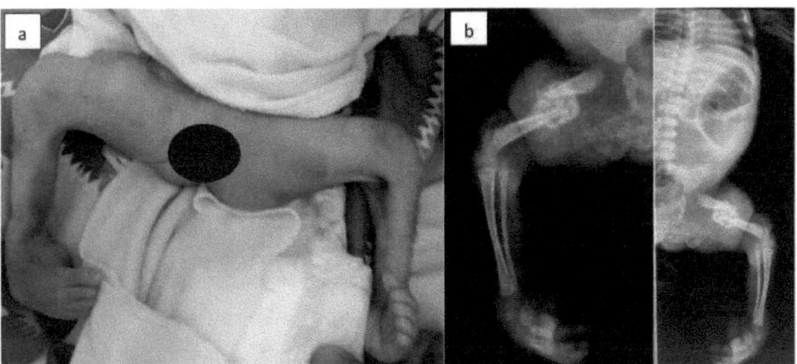

Figure N°43: BRUCK syndrome a- Morphological aspect b- Radiological aspect

VII.5.3.3 Secondary demineralization :

These demineralizations can be iatrogenic (corticoid, heparin, methotrexate, chemotherapy, anticonvulsant), deficiency-related (vitamin D deficiency, vitamin C deficiency, etc.).
copper....), due to vitamin-resistant rickets, of endocrine origin (type I diabetes, hypothyroidism, hypogonadism, cushing's disease), of digestive origin (gastrointestinal disease, etc.), or due to a combination of these.
celiac disease, chronic inflammatory bowel disease, intestinal malabsorption), nephropathic, hematopathic, leukemic and other cancers. Hypertrophic callus in osteogenesis imperfecta type V may be confused with osteosarcoma [70], [120], [121].

VIII. MEDICAL CARE:

Osteogenesis imperfecta must be managed by a specialized multidisciplinary team coordinated by a competent reference center.

During the paediatric period, it is essentially organized around the central pivot:

- Orthopedic surgeons (treatment of fractures and deformities of the limbs and spine).
- The paediatrician (treatment of chronic or post-fracture pain and medical treatment mainly with bisphosphonates).
- The specialist in physical medicine and rehabilitation (re-education, adaptation).
- Geneticists (research and genetic counseling).

Many healthcare professionals are involved in the overall care of patients: The anesthetist, pain specialist, ENT doctor, pulmonologist, rheumatologist, radiologist, cardiologist, neurosurgeon, dental surgeon, stomatologist, masseur-physiotherapist, orthoprosthetist and dental technician, occupational therapist, psychologist and social worker.

VIII.   1. Family and parental education :

Care of the family and the sick child must be the first step in multidisciplinary management [122], [123].

At birth, parents need to be familiar with this pathology, with existing therapeutic methods, and receive training in how to behave towards their child. They must learn how to position, handle and transport their baby.

Handling must be gentle, avoiding all prohibited gestures that may cause fractures.

Positioning should promote the child's alignment, using soft calluses.

You need :

- Use a headrest that relieves pressure on the cephalic areas to avoid brachycephaly and plagiocephaly.
- Place children in supine position, protecting them with rolls of cloth to keep the trunk straight and avoid thoracic and spinal deformities.
- Focus on stretching the lower limbs to protect the child from vicious hip flexion.
- Lay the car seat flat and move children in horizontal strollers.
- Ensure their child's hygiene by bathing in a standard baby bathtub,

with the child stabilized inside by wedges on the sides.

When it comes to clothing, cotton should be used, as the use of synthetic garments increases sweating in these children, which can be a source of hydroelectrolytic imbalance.

Teach parents to develop their children's cognitive side by stimulating them with appropriate games and activities.

At a slightly older age, parents need to be trained to manage pain, immobilize a fracture, stimulate the patient's physical activity and keep multidisciplinary consultation appointments.

In the case of children, we need to teach them to live with their pathology, avoid untimely movements that can lead to fractures, and engage in appropriate physical activity to preserve their muscular and bone capital. They need to be reassured and reassured by stimulating physical activity.

They need to learn how to combat pain, maintain joint mobility and master safe transfer and movement techniques.

It makes more sense to restore their self-confidence by encouraging them to take part in regular, appropriate physical activity, participate in social activities and schooling, and introduce them into social circles as fully-fledged children. Self-confidence is the only guarantee that they will adhere to their treatment, and thus enjoy a better quality of life.

VIII. 2. Re-education and functional rehabilitation:

The aim of physical medicine and rehabilitation is to improve the functional capabilities of patients suffering from osteogenesis imperfecta. It is indicated for all forms of osteogenesis imperfecta, and is the only treatment for mild forms.

It combines work in specialized rehabilitation centers with support from local physiotherapists [63] [122], [123], [124].

Rehabilitation aims to prevent immobility-induced bone loss, strengthen overall muscular strength, optimize functional independence and ensure autonomy, socialization and quality of life.

Re-education should help children with osteogenesis imperfecta to stand upright, and provide them with good muscle trophicity, a better way to offset skeletal fragility.

Respiratory physiotherapy is essential, especially for patients with thoracic and spinal development disorders and intrinsic lung parenchyma damage.

Orthoses play a limited role in the management of OI. They are used to stabilize lax joints (e.g. ankle and subtalar joints) and to prevent progressive deformities and fractures [63] [122], [123], [124].

Prolonged immobilization is contraindicated, as it is a source of bone loss. It should be light and of short duration. It can be made with plaster, preferably with resin, and even better with flexible resin.

Immobilization with plaster, resin or orthoses must be adapted to the patient's functional state. These devices can be used as post-operative restraints, as support material during rehabilitation, and as protection during patient transport.

It is more important to provide walking aids, specialized wheelchairs and home adaptation devices to improve the patient's mobility and function at home.

It's important to remember the role of post-operative rehabilitation, which consists of early, protected and progressive care of the patient. It must ensure effective functional rehabilitation of unlimited duration, the only guarantee of functional autonomy. Social integration depends on the degree of this autonomy [63] [122], [123], [124].

Rehabilitation must focus on "MAKE THE patient MOVE", whatever the form of the pathology. We need to work on ambulation, muscle strengthening and proprioceptivity. Children must be trained to exercise in "Sport and Disability" consultations, so that sports activities can be adapted to the patient [125].

The use of certain equipment such as Whole Body Vibration helps to increase muscle and bone mass [126].

VIII.   3. Medical treatment:

In osteogenesis imperfecta, it is argued that there is an imbalance between bone formation and resorption. Bone formation is insufficient, and the close relationship between osteoblasts and osteoclasts leads to a secondary increase in bone resorption [26], [50]. The result is an increased risk of fracture from childhood onwards, which must be prevented and treated. Several treatments are available to reduce fracture risk, either by reducing osteoclastic activity or by stimulating osteoblastic activity.

At present, there is no evidence that these molecules prevent long-bone deformities or slow the progression of spinal deformities.

The most widely used molecules are bisphosphonates (Aredia, Actonel, Fosamax, Bonviva, Aclasta).

Bisphosphonates (BP) were introduced in 1987 by NAGANT DE DEUXCHAISNES and DEVOGLAER [8], who offered them to a child with osteogenesis imperfecta, with the aim of increasing bone density and mass to prevent fractures. This molecule had proved its efficacy in the treatment of postmenopausal and cortisone-induced osteoporosis, with encouraging effects. Since then, several studies have been carried out on this molecule [8].

BPs are analogues of pyrophosphates, with the P-O-P bond replaced by a P-C-P bond. The most recent BPs, such as pamidronate, neridronate, risedronate or zoledronate, have a nitrogen atom in a side chain, inhibiting the metabolic pathway of mevalonate; this induces a decrease in bone resorption through reduced osteoclastic activity and accelerated osteoclastic apoptosis.

The PB molecule does not cure the disease, but acts by reducing bone resorption, thus enabling bone densification. Its administration requires a clinical, radiological, densitometric and biological assessment prior to each course of treatment [127].

Since GLORIEUX's first study in 1998 [128], antiresorptive treatment of osteogenesis imperfecta with bisphosphonates (BP) has become the only pharmacological treatment option for moderate to severe osteogenesis imperfecta.

Subsequently, numerous studies [128], [129], [130] have demonstrated the positive effect of BP on bone mineral density (BMD). Recently, two studies have shown a reduction in fractures in young children, while preserving their linear growth [129], [130] [131].

In all cases, an adequate level of vitamin D (25(OH) D3) is necessary for a good response to BP [132], [133].

As a general rule, BPs are well tolerated, but their administration may be accompanied by a series of undesirable effects that are not entirely risk-free (Table No. 05).

Category	Undesirable effect	Prevention / treatment

Acute, immediately after infusion	hypocalcemia	Adequate daily intake of calcium and vitamin D. 0-6 years: 500mg Ca. After 6 years/ 100mg Ca
Acute, 24 to 48 hours after first dose	Flu-like syndrome	Paracetamol 15-20 mg /kg/dose every 6 hours
	Bronchospasm in infants under one year of age	Monitoring, salbutamol
Bones	Remodeling disorder	
	Possible adverse effect on bone growth	
	Reduced remodeling	
	Possible delay in the fracture healing process	
other	Weight gain	
	Uveitis	
	Renal failure after high-dose bisphosphonates	
	Pregnancy: influence on the fetus	Pregnancy testing for post-menarche girls and women, contraception
	Osteonecrosis of the jaw	Probably not significant with osteogenesis imperfecta

Table N°05: Adverse effects of bisphosphonate treatment [27].

The decision to start treatment with bisphosphonates is based on clinical and/or radiological arguments, not densitometry. Bisphosphonate treatment is discussed in cases of at least two fractures, at different sites, in the previous year, such as vertebral compression with or without spinal statics disorders (scoliosis or kyphosis); or in severe neonatal forms, particularly in children with ante- and perinatal fractures. The decision to discontinue treatment should be discussed at least once a year, if possible during multidisciplinary consultations.

No bisphosphonate has been approved for use in children with osteogenesis imperfecta. The decision to treat children with osteogenesis imperfecta with bisphosphonates, and their place in the therapeutic strategy, must be taken after medical and surgical consultation involving orthopedic surgeons, bone pathology specialists, physical and rehabilitation medicine specialists and pediatric endocrinologists.

Currently, the recommended duration of treatment is 2 to 4 years, depending on the severity of osteogenesis imperfecta, stability of clinical condition and bone density [23] [26], [27], [63].

The indication for maintenance treatment will be based on changes in bone densitometry, bone remodelling markers and fracture incidence [23] [26], [27], [63].

Cure of PB is discussed in surgical practice. According to some authors [134], PB should be discontinued one week before surgery and until the consolidation callus is visualized.

BPs are implicated in high bone densification, a source of iatrogenic osteopetrosis (Figure N°43-a), with the risk of bone rigidity and fractures, remodeling disorders and delayed consolidation of fractures and osteotomies, or even pseudarthrosis (Figure N°43-b). It is advisable to keep surgery away from periods of BP intake [28], [135], [136].

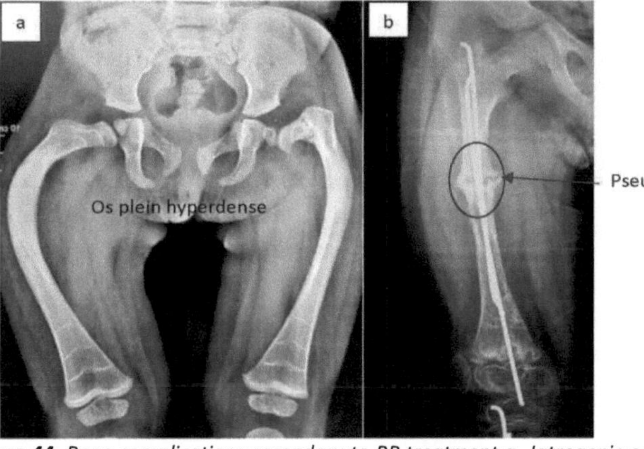

Figure 44: Bone complications secondary to BP treatment a- Iatrogenic osteopetrosis b-Pseudarthrosis

Thanks to the development of current research, other molecules are being introduced:

Denosumab (anti-RANK ligand monoclonal antibody; prolia) has been introduced in certain recessive forms of osteogenesis imperfecta that respond poorly to BP. This molecule reduces fracture frequency, increases bone mineral density and improves patient mobility [65].

Bone formation stimulators, such as teriparatide (Forsteo) and other molecules such as anticathepsin K, a bone resorber, or the anti-sclerostin antibody, are on the way. The latter, thanks to its potential to increase bone remodeling tenfold by reducing resorption and stimulating bone formation. This molecule is an ideal candidate for the treatment of osteogenesis imperfecta [23].

For these new molecules, there are insufficient data to assess their ability to reduce fracture risk; nevertheless, studies in mice are very promising [136]. Other gene and cell therapies (marrow transplants) are modern methods currently being evaluated [137].

Tomorrow's medicine will enable us to choose the right molecule for the genetic mutation. If the patient suffers from osteogenesis imperfecta, where the bone-forming pathway is primarily responsible for bone fragility, we will propose a treatment that stimulates it [64].

VIII.   4. Intensive care anesthesia :

Anesthetic management of children with osteogenesis imperfecta remains a challenge. It can lead to serious complications.

Because of their bone fragility, intraoperative manipulations such as abrupt movements, intubation maneuvers and even the BP cuff, expose these patients to the risk of fractures. What's more, apart from bone, osteogenesis imperfecta affects all organs, so there is also a risk of respiratory, cardiac and hemorrhagic decompensation in these patients.

All anaesthetic procedures should therefore benefit from prior preparation, and respiratory and cardiac function should be explored:

- Respiratory function testing (RFT), as a minimum, is useful in moderate and severe forms of osteogenesis imperfecta with large thoracic and spinal deformities. It should be performed from the age of 5 in all children with vertebral compression.
- Cardiac ultrasound is usually required for patients aged 10 and over.

The biological work-up should include a double blood grouping determination, a blood count formula, a haemostasis work-up with a platelet function study using the Platelet Function Analyser to determine platelet occlusion time, especially if there is a history of haemorrhage.

An electrolyte balance is necessary because of the increased risk of water and electrolyte losses and ketosis in children with osteogenesis imperfecta, particularly in severe forms requiring long operating times.

Intraoperatively, the difficulty lies in:

- Taking venous lines from vessels that are often fragile.
- At intubation, the anatomy of the respiratory tree is sometimes modified, and the dental arches are fragile.
- The risk of neurological disorders due to the fragility of the cervical hinge, which, although rare, are still serious because they can be life-threatening.
- For this reason, it is advisable to take the following precautions:
- Gently manipulate the patient, especially during positioning and intubation.
- Place several approaches to avoid the risk of bleeding.

In all cases, for severe forms, locoregional anesthesia is always preferable to general anesthesia, especially if intubation is difficult.

Epidural anaesthesia or spinal anaesthesia (figure N°45) are possible if the patient has no arthrodesis material in the spine.

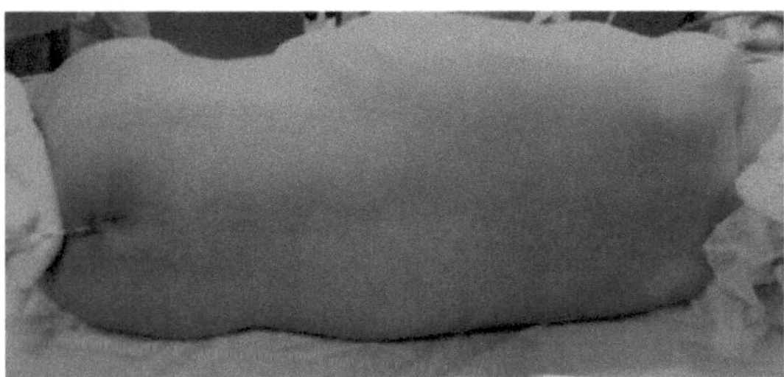

Figure 45: Preoperative view of caudal anesthesia in a patient undergoing surgery for osteogenesis imperfecta Severe form [personal collection].

Ultrasound-guided anesthesia (figure 46) and peripheral nerve blocks are associated with low morbidity.

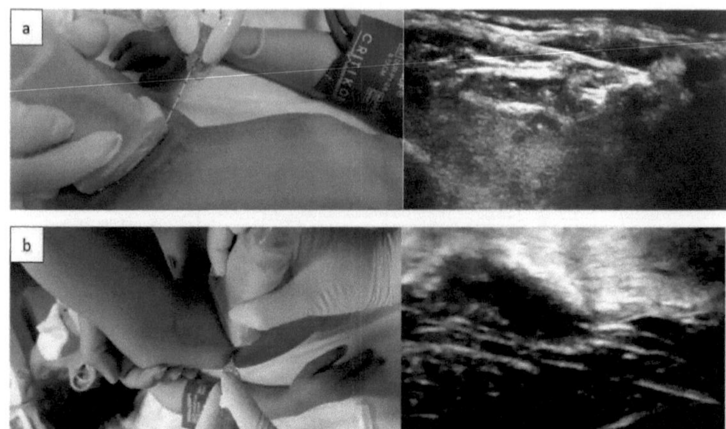

Figure 46: Ultrasound-guided locoregional anesthesia [personal collection] a- Ultrasound-guided location and injection for femoral block b- Ultrasound-guided location and injection for sciatic block

Locoregional anaesthesia offers greater safety, analgesia and prolonged postoperative comfort for the patient. Nevertheless, there is a risk of complications: ROTHSCHILD et al [80] found in a series of 205 anaesthesia cases that intubation was difficult in 1.5% of cases, 1% of children had rib and humerus fractures caused by the monitoring cuff, it was difficult to take a venous line in 4% of cases, and blood loss with clinical repercussions was found in 17% of cases. Post-operative cardiovascular and metabolic complications were mentioned but not assessed. These complications are most frequent in severe cases.

Type III osteogenesis imperfecta had a 95% chance of complications compared with type I

Due to repeated surgery, children with osteogenesis imperfecta undergo frequent anesthetic exposure, and the likelihood of encountering problems depends essentially on the severity of the case. Nevertheless, meticulous preparation, full knowledge of the difficulties encountered and the means of anticipating them, together with adequate management, should make the procedure safe [138].

In the postoperative period, resuscitation must be concerned with :

- Post-operative analgesia, the development of new analgesic molecules, the use of morphine pumps and, above all, the generalization of locoregional analgesia have revolutionized pain management in osteogenesis imperfecta. It is important to note the role of the paramedic, who must master the handling of these patients and provide them with the best possible comfort.

- Fluid and electrolyte balance through controlled filling and blood transfusion, and daily monitoring of hemoglobin levels for the first 4 days after multiple osteotomies.

Despite advances in medical management, anesthesia and resuscitation, these children still run the risk of death at birth, in childhood or in adulthood. ALLCON and PETERSON [93] have summarized the causes of death in Table N°06.

Causes of death	osteogenesis imperfecta type III	osteogenesis imperfecta type I - IV	total
Respiratory causes	08	22	30
Spinal cord compression		3	03
Bronchopulmonary infection	29	13	42
Inhalation pneumonitis		01	01
Acute respiratory failure		01	01
Chronic respiratory insufficiency		01	01
Cardiorespiratory failure	01		01

Table N°06: *Causes of death in osteogenesis imperfecta [93].*

In addition to these most frequent causes, others have been incriminated, namely neoplastic, digestive, metabolic, endocrine and nutritional causes [139].

Even if the management of these patients is now well codified, the means more elaborate and the techniques more developed, the complexity of these cases means that complications cannot be completely avoided [140].

IX. SURGICAL MANAGEMENT:

IX. 1. General information on palliative osteosynthesis of long bones :

Osteogenesis imperfecta is both a constitutional and acquired condition, combining bone fragility, recurrent fractures and skeletal deformities. The frequent immobilization of these patients leads to osteopenia, which only exacerbates the disease. For these reasons, surgery must provide effective protection against fragility, prevent diaphyseal deformities and minimize the occurrence of fractures. Surgery remains an important palliative means in the chain of therapeutic management of osteogenesis imperfecta [15], [29].

Rigid segmental osteosynthesis alone (Fig. N°47), limited to a diaphyseal portion, is a source of fracture above or below the fixture through mechanical impingement. It is therefore banned from the osteosynthesis arsenal for osteogenesis imperfecta fractures. Occasionally, this type of osteosynthesis may be indicated, provided it is combined with centromedullary protection [29].

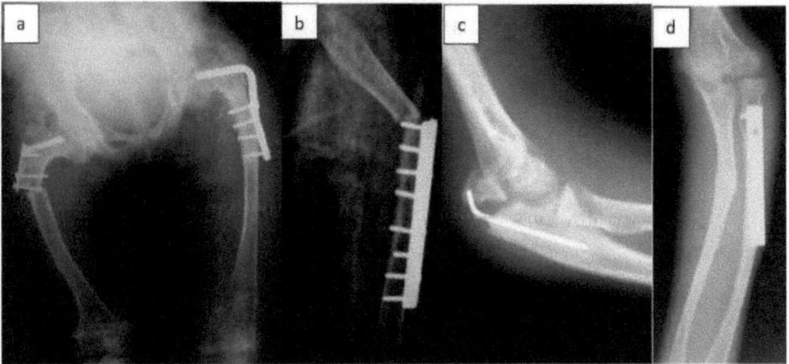

Figure N°47: Radiographs illustrating segmental osteosynthesis [personal collection]: a: fracture under a catherinette, b: fracture above a femoral plate c: broaching of the olecranon, d: radial plate

The osteosynthesis device must be lightweight, can be fixed to the bone by screw fixation on either side of the nail or centromedullary pins, and can be secured by unicortical screws or cerclage wires [143].

Since the first publications by SOFIELD [9], palliative osteosynthesis using internal stents has opened the door to current surgical principles in this pathology. Since then, centromedullary nailing of the long bones has been the method of choice for treating fractures and deformities in children with osteogenesis imperfecta.

However, SOFIELD's single tutor [9] poses two major problems to overcome:
- The small size of the bones means that small, thin, flexible nails offer little protection.
- Growth: single, non-telescopic nails become too short after around 2 years of growth, generating the risk of fracture "at the nail ends" in unprotected areas (figure N°48).

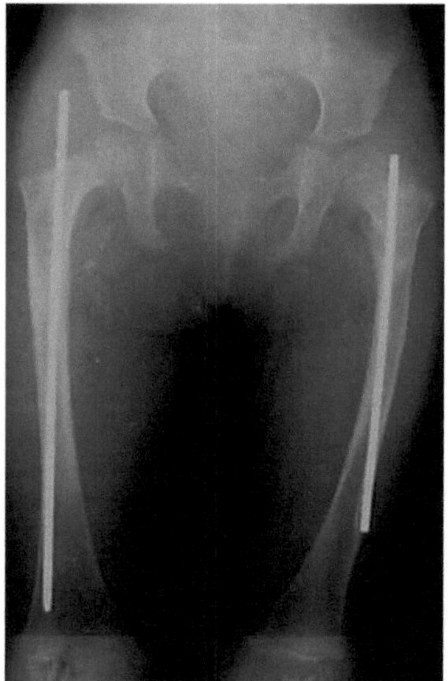

Figure 48: X-ray of two femurs treated with a single non-expandable nail (SOFIELD method) [Personal collection].

The principle of the single nail has undergone technical progress, revolutionizing surgery for osteogenesis imperfecta thanks to the contribution of modern radiology techniques and the development of closed-focus nailing and pinning techniques [141].
BAILEY and DUBOW introduced the telescopic nail in 1963 [11], [142].

In 1987 [12], METAIZEAU demonstrated the results of stable elastic centromedullary pinning and sliding or telescopic pinning of long bones in the treatment of fractures and deformities in osteogenesis imperfecta.

Thanks to these revolutions, we have moved from extensive sub-periosteal exposure of the diaphyses, multiple osteotomies and alignment of the bone on a single inextensible nail to less aggressive techniques limiting the importance of surgical approaches, reducing the extent of de-periostealization and using material that can be extended during growth.

IX. 2. Purpose of palliative long-bone osteosynthesis:

The aims of osteosynthesis in this growing population with fragile and often deformed bone are to:

- Strengthen this bone and provide effective protection against bone fragility.
- Protect long bones during growth.
- Realign long bones.
- Prevent long-bone deformities and minimize fracture frequency and displacement.
- Enable early and lasting functional rehabilitation.

The aim is to help patients regain their comfort and independence, enabling them to return to school and social life (figure N°49).

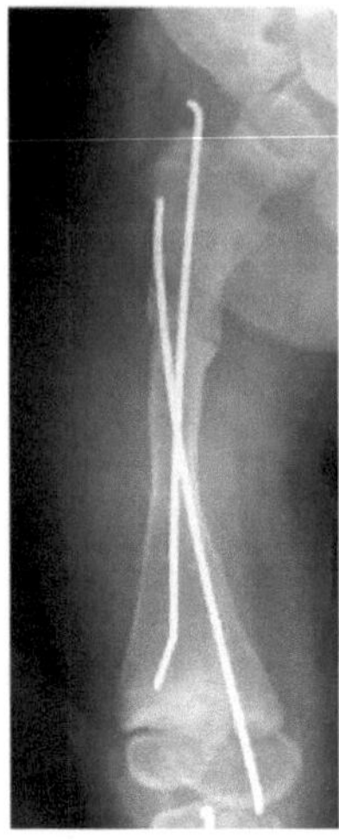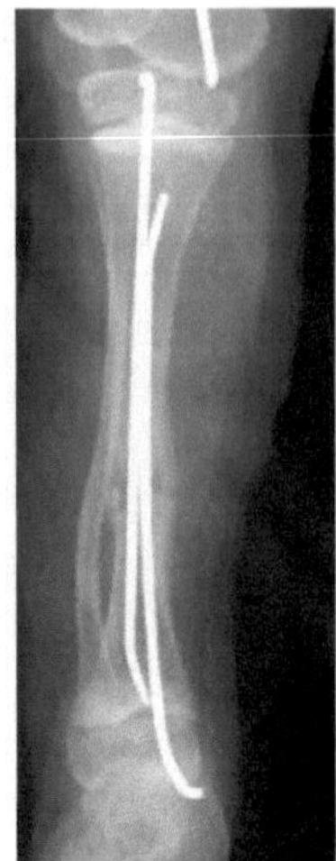

Figure 49: Femur and leg X-ray with telescopic mounting for diaphyseal protection during growth [personal collection].

IX. 3. Biomechanical principles:

A wide range of osteosynthesis devices are currently available, including telescopic nails, pins, plates, screws and cerclage wires.

Regardless of the osteosynthesis material used, the most important thing is to be familiar with the particularities of osteogenesis imperfecta, to master the know-how for each technique, to establish the indication, and to identify and manage the complications that may arise in the post-operative period [143].

The basic principle is to protect the entire diaphysis, from one epiphysis to the other. This is easy for the tibia, humerus and both forearm bones, but less obvious for the femur. For the femur, the diaphysis and femoral neck must be protected at the same time [143].

In particular, correct diaphyseal alignment must be achieved in the frontal plane without varus or valgus and without deviation in the sagittal plane.

In the lower limb, this alignment must ensure that the neck of the femur remains in valgus and that the knee line is horizontal from the front and the side [143].

Implant insertion must be atraumatic with respect to the growth plate, to minimize the risk of iatrogenic epiphysiodesis. Care must be taken not to induce rotational anomalies postoperatively, and patients must be immobilized in correct positions for short periods.

Regardless of the osteosynthesis material used, excessively bulky material should be avoided to prevent progressive bone resorption [143].

When replacing hardware, preference should be given to replacement with a thinner nail than the first, or outright replacement by simple pinning to minimize cortical bone resorption [143].

IX.   4. Surgical methods and techniques :

All patients must have a high-quality preoperative radiological workup to enable analysis of the various deformities and preparation of the osteosynthesis material.

All intramedullary stenting techniques are radiosurgical.

An image intensifier must be available in the operating room to guide the introduction and placement of osteosynthesis material, and to define the site of corrective osteotomies. X-rays are also used to monitor the implant's progress through the sometimes sinuous bone. These difficulties expose both patient and practitioner to considerable radiation exposure.

IX.4.1. Telescopic nailing:

SOFIELD [9] was the first to introduce the principle of centromedullary nailing in osteogenesis imperfecta. This technique used a single, inextensible nail that did not protect the bone during growth and had to be changed during these phases [144]. This technique led to deformities and fractures at the distal ends of the nail. This method has now been abandoned.

IX.4.1.1. The BAILEY and DUBOW nail

In 1963, BAILEY and DUBOW [11], [142] introduced the telescopic nail (figure N°50).

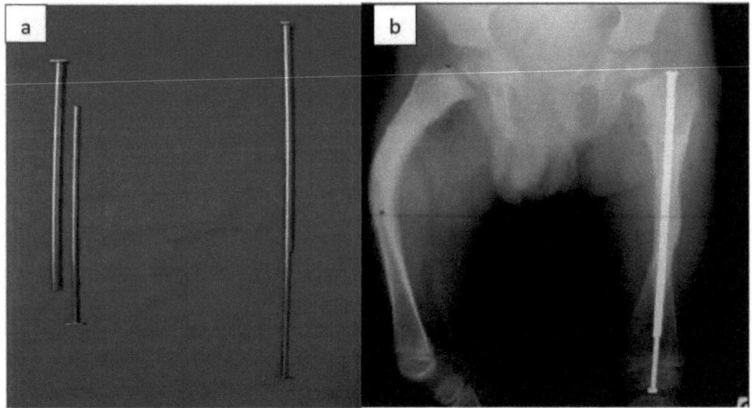

Figure N°50: *BAILEY-DUBOS nail [collection of G. FINIDORI] a- Parts of the Bailley-Dubow nail b- Left intra femoral Bailley-Dubow nail*

This nail consists of :

- A perforated cylindrical tubular female part with a thread inside one of its ends and a T-piece that can be screwed into this female part and crimped into the bone.
- A solid male part, threaded at one end
- to which another T-piece is screwed.

The male part slides inside the female cylinder.

In the classic technique, the nail was used for centromedullary drilling. Nowadays, the telescopic nail is supplied with an ancillary comprising a long, more rigid drill bit of slightly larger diameter than the nail. This bit can be used as a guide. The ancillary also provides a second nail guide.

The length and diameter of the nail must be determined preoperatively. For each patient, the nail dimensions are based on radiological calculations performed on front and side views centered on the maximum deformity. This requires accurate enlargement of the X-ray. However, this calculation remains difficult and approximate. These sizes vary from one individual to another, especially as the bone is often elliptical [145].

This telescopic nail is only available in five different diameters. It must be prepared before each operation to avoid any intraoperative modifications. Such modifications could lead to problems such as mismatching the male and female parts of the nail, blocking the telescoping system and corroding the material.

Telescopic nailing frequently requires a joint approach (shoulder, elbow, knee and ankle), which can be detrimental from a functional point of view, especially for the ankle [29].

In the femur [29]:
A guide drill is pulled upwards under fluoroscopic control through a small incision under the patella and a small incision in the patellar tendon.
Penetration of the drill bit takes place at the bottom of the inter-condylar notch, in a direction perpendicular to the knee joint line.
The drill bit is retracted intramedullarily and, whenever it comes up against a cortical bone, the diaphysis must be realigned, either by osteoclasia, percutaneous osteotomy or mini-approach.
As many osteotomies as necessary must be performed to align the shaft, ensuring that the femoral neck is in valgus.
Once the femur is aligned with the guide drill perpendicular to the knee joint and the neck in valgus, this drill is brought out at the outer edge of the neck and percutaneously at buttock level, placing the hip in adduction and flexion.
The female part is then screwed to the distal end of the guide bit, and progressively moved up into the femur and buttock outside the skin planes. The first T-piece is screwed onto the female part, then impacted and crimped at the upper edge of the neck medial to the greater trochanter. The male part is then inserted into the female part, and impacted into the distal epiphysis of the femur with its second T-piece.

On the tibia [29]:
The guide wire is introduced via a mini lateral para-patellar approach, through a bony penetration point in the center of the tibial plateaus, anterior to the insertion of the cruciate ligament. The guide drill progresses in the same way as for the femur, down to the distal epiphysis. The fibula is not usually approached, as it is fragile and can be corrected by manipulating the tibia. Introduction of the female part requires an anterolateral arthrotomy of the tibiotalar joint space, after tilting the talus medially and posteriorly. The guide drill is replaced by the nail, as for the femur.

Positioning the telescopic nail in the leg is difficult. It is difficult to position the nail correctly, as it is often placed anteriorly, and distal epiphyseal fixation is very delicate. Arthrotomy and manipulation of the nail often result in joint damage.

In the humerus [29]:

The principle remains the same. The entire upper limb is prepared, shoulder free.

Through a short posterior approach to the elbow, giving access to the coronoid fossa and lateral condyle, the guide drill is introduced from the lateral condyle slightly outside the olecranon to avoid stiffening the elbow. The guide drill is withdrawn into the proximal end of the humerus under fluoroscopic control, just anterior to the acromion. Nail placement is identical to that for the femur and tibia.

It is difficult to position the nail correctly in the humerus, and humeral deviation into ulna varus is often induced.

Apart from femoral, tibial and humeral nailing, there are no indications for telescopic forearm nailing in children with osteogenesis imperfecta.
Post-operative immobilization is ensured with a Mayo-Clinic bandage, taking care to avoid rotatory disorders.

The management of osteogenesis imperfecta has evolved over time. Severe forms have become less frequent in developed countries; patients are operated on for fragility and less severe diaphyseal deformities. It has therefore become logical to envisage less invasive procedures, with fewer complications.

IX.4.1.2. Variants of telescopic nails :

IX.4.1.2.1. The SHEFFIELD nail:

The SHEFFIELD nail [146] (figure N°51) is a BAILLY and DUBOW nail for which SHEFFIELD modified the T-piece attachment.
This T-piece, which was removable and screwed into the old BAILLY DUBOW nail, has become a T-piece attached to the ends of the male and female parts of this new telescopic nail.

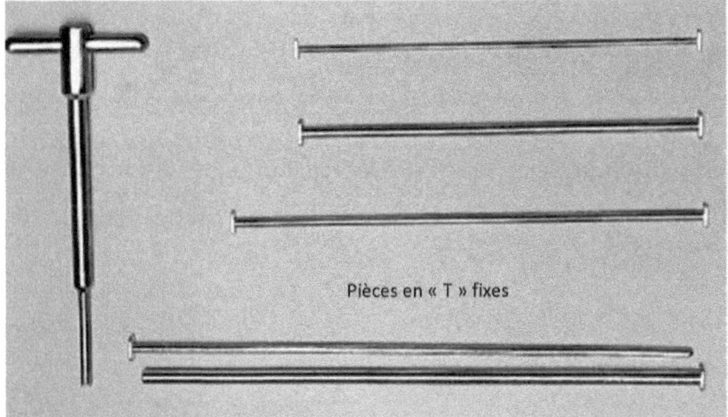

Figure 51: SHEFFIELD nail [146].

IX.4.1.2.2. BAILEY and DUBOW nail modified by FINIDORI:

For a long time, the team at Necker Enfants Malades [29] remained faithful to the classic nail of BAILEY and DUBOW, except that to facilitate the impaction of the male part of the classic nail, GEORGE FINIDORIE added a notch on the distal part of the male part to stabilize the male part impaction during its intraosseous impaction (figure N°52).

This same team hardly ever uses nailing in the tibia any more, preferring sliding pinning, which is simpler to perform and less invasive.

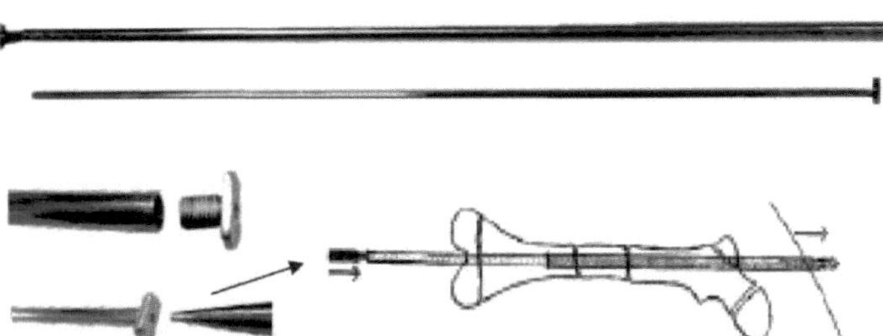

Figure 52: Modification of the impaction point of the male part of the Bailey-Dubow nail [29].

IX.4.1.2.3. The FASSIER DUVAL nail:

The FASSIER DUVAL nail [147], [148], [149] consists of two parts: a solid male part, threaded at its distal end, and a hollow cylindrical female part, threaded at its proximal end (figure N°53 - a).

Introduced in 2000, this nail was initially used for femur nailing in children suffering from osteogenesis imperfecta. Thanks to the results obtained, the indication for this nail was extended to the leg (fig. N°53-b, N°54), the humerus and other pathologies such as fibrous dysplasia.

The main advantage of this nail is that, compared with the BAILEY and DUBOW nails, no arthrotomy is required for its insertion, as it is introduced via a single retrograde route.

Its use requires a technical platform comprising a radiolucent operating table, an image intensifier, Pega-médical FD ancillary equipment and a Midas-rex system for intraoperative nail cutting.

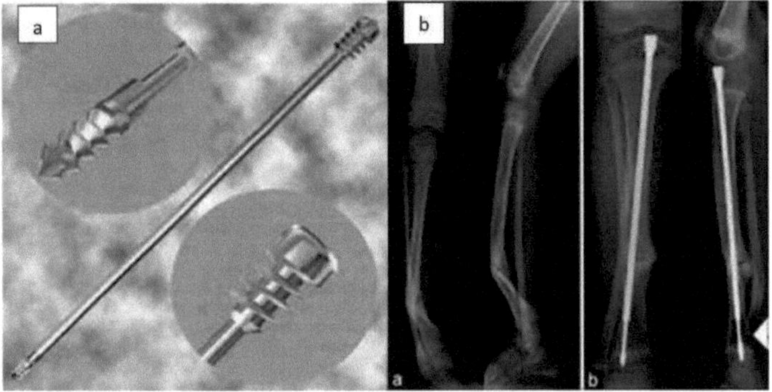

Figure N°53: image illustrating the Fassier-Duval nail [149].
a- Image of the components of the Fassier-Duval nail
b- X-ray of a telescopic centromedullary nailing of the leg with an F-D nail

This nail must be prepared before each operation. Length and diameter are measured on good-quality, full-size front and side views.

The diameter of the nail is that of the female part and corresponds to the diameter of the narrowest part of the medullary canal.

The length of the nail is calculated from a profile shot. It corresponds to the length of the female part. The measurement corresponds to the distance between the proximal epiphysis and the distal growth plate, from which we subtract the subtraction wedge dimensions to be made when aligning the bone, plus 7 mm from the threaded end of the male part.

The nail is inserted from distal to proximal. The centromedullary path is prepared by reaming, using progressive diameter reamers on the nail guide and under fluoroscopic control. The reaming diameter is 2mm greater than that of the pre-prepared female part. This reaming is stopped a few millimeters before the growth plate.

Using a nail guide, the male part is inserted from top to bottom under radiological control. The distal end is screwed into the distal epiphysis in a single operation, to avoid damaging the growth plate. Care must be taken to ensure that the screw is in the center of the epiphysis. The guide nail is removed, and the male part is held in place with a special device supplied with the insertion ancillary, to avoid tearing the growth plate and causing epiphysiodesis.

The female nail is then pushed onto the male nail from proximal to distal, then fixed and screwed into the proximal epiphysis with its proximal end. A hexagonal screwdriver is used until the threaded part of the female part is embedded in the epiphysis.
The proximal end of the protruding male part is cut flush with the female part, avoiding damage to the cutting edge which could prevent the nail from sliding.

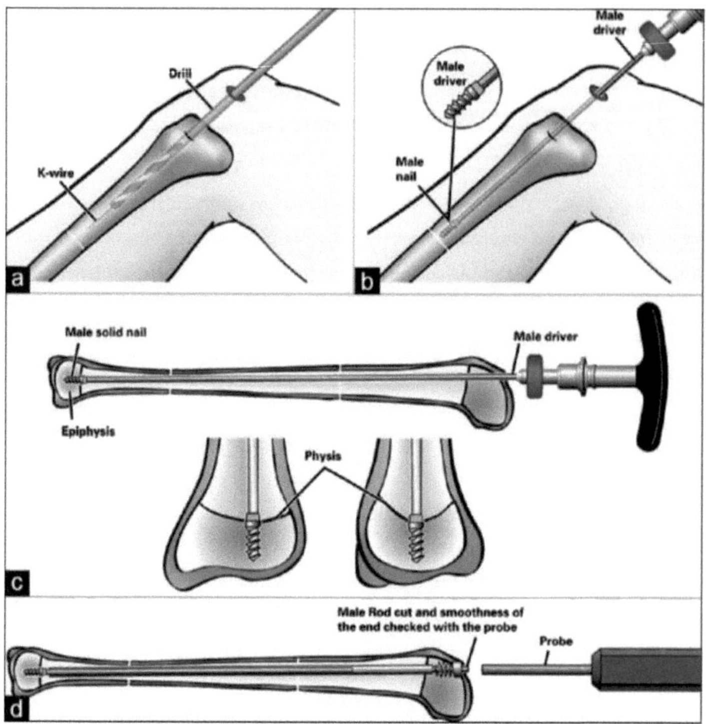

*Figure 54: Diagram of the various stages of leg nailing with an F- telescopic nail.
D [147]: a: reaming of diaphyseal shaft - b: introduction of male part - c: distal intra-
epiphyseal screwing of male part - d: introduction and fixation of female part.*

IX.4.1.2.4. The DMM nail: Nail For epiphisary attachment without opening the Joints

This type of nailing is based on the same principles as conventional telescopic nails. Its distinctive feature is a female part with a flattened tip at the distal end, housing a locking hole, and a male part with an L-shaped, perforated proximal end. The female part is locked by a pin placed intraepiphyseally under radiological control using a special sighting device. The nail is inserted via an ascending approach. The nail is introduced via a single proximal route. The female part is introduced from the proximal to the distal epiphysis, under radiological control. Once the distal part of the female part has been introduced into the distal epiphysis of the bone, it is locked by an epiphyseal pin introduced with the aiming device from inside to outside into the locking hole. The male part is slid into the female part from top to bottom, then fixed through its curved part into the bone, either with a non-absorbable thread or with a locking pin (Fig. N°55).

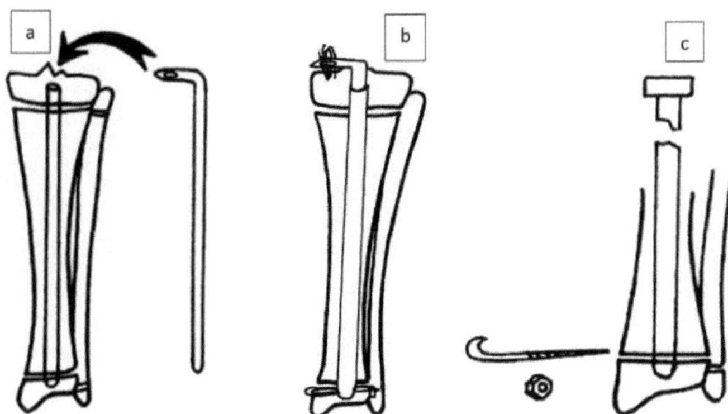

Figure 55: *Diagram illustrating a DMM nail a- Nail insertion steps b- Proximal fixation of the male part c- Distal fixation of the female part*

IX.4.1.2.5. The telescopic nail modified by Tae-Joon Cho:

The TAE-JOON CHO nail [150] is not too different from the DMM nail. It follows the same principle of use. It has a single point of introduction, via a proximal approach. The female part is identical to that of BAILEY and DUBOW, except that it has a fixed T-shaped proximal end. The male part has a flattened, perforated end.

The female part is inserted first, up to the distal conjugation cartilage, then fixed at the neck- greater trochanter junction. The male part is inserted into the female part from top to bottom, with the distal end passing through the CC under radiological control. A locking pin is inserted into the distal epiphysis, passing through the locking hole in the male part from lateral to medial (Fig. N°56).

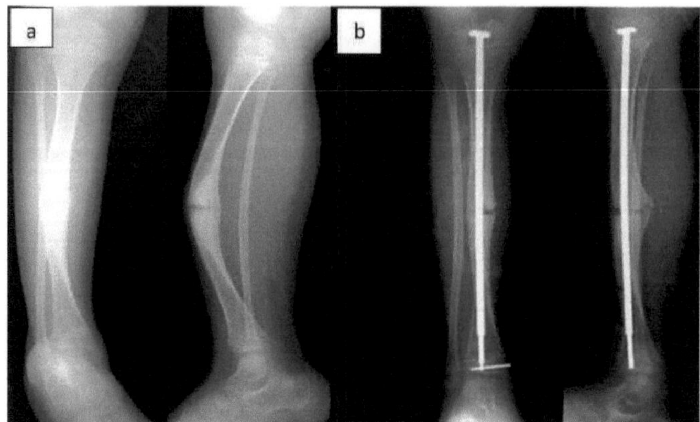

Figure N°56: telescopic nail modified by Tae-Joon Cho et al [150] a- Preoperative radiographs of the 2 leg bones b- Postoperative radiograph with telescopic nailing

IX.4.1.2.6. The HIMEX extensible nail:

The HIMEX nail is identical in design to the BAILEY and DUBOW nail. W.D. BELANGERO et al [151] have modified the ends of the male and female parts. They removed the T-pieces and replaced them with hooks which they drove into the bone (Fig. N°57).

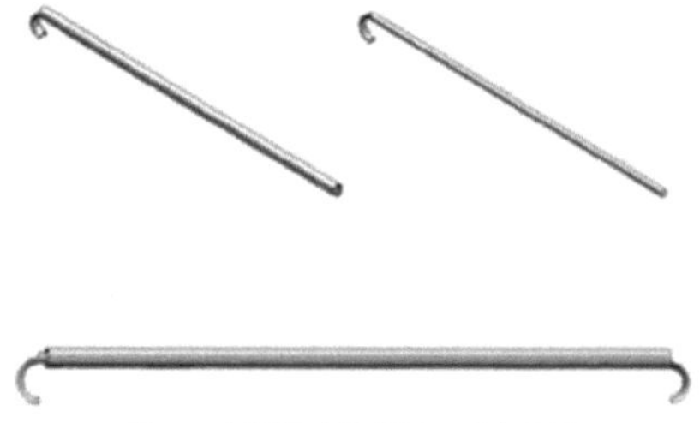

Figure N°57: HIMEX nail [151]

IX.4.1.2.7. Corkscrew tipped telescopic nail:

This nail is identical to the FASSIER DUVALE nail, and its installation technique is the same. The difference between these two nails is in the distal part of the male part. The Corkscrew tipped telescopic nail [152] has a corkscrew-shaped end. This corkscrew shape is said to be less invasive than the threaded end of the FASSIER DUVAL nail. According to these users, this nail is less traumatic for the growth plate. For these authors, this type of nail has fewer disadvantages than the classic nail. It requires a single point of penetration, there is less joint aggression, especially at the distal end of the tibia, and there is less debricolage of the implant. These nails are mainly used for the femur and tibia.

IX.4.2. Sliding or telescopic spindles :

In 1987, METAIZEAU JP introduced the concept of stable elastic sliding centromedullary pinning for the management of osteogenesis imperfecta. He recommended replacing the telescopic nail with two pins, one descending, the other ascending, sliding one on top of the other in the shaft [12].
It is flexible, less rigid and less expensive than the telescopic nail [153].
This technique requires MAITEZEAU wires. These are wires curved at the ends, with different diameters and lengths. Alternatively, stainless steel Kirchner wires can be used. These are minimally invasive and reliable [29].
Advances in intraoperative radiology have facilitated the use of this technique. It is a radiosurgical technique.

IX.4.2.1. Centromedullary telescopic sliding pinning:

This consists of placing a metal stent consisting of two wires, which are positioned in such a way as to ensure bone support during growth (Fig. N°58). The first is inserted down the bone, with its proximal end anchored in the proximal epiphysis. The second ascending along the operated bone, with its distal end anchored in the distal epiphysis. Thanks to their epiphyseal anchorage, these pins will slide over each other during growth, ensuring their long-term protective role.

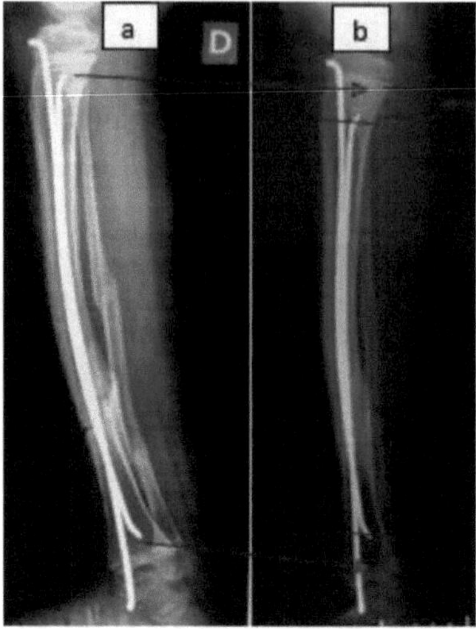

Figure 58: Centromedullary telescopic leg pinning [personal collection] a- X-ray at 45 days post-op b- X-ray at 6 months post-op

Humeral level:

The first pin is anchored distally in the lateral condyle, pushed up to just below the proximal growth plate via a percutaneous incision and under radiological control. The second wire is lowered through a small percutaneous incision located one fingerbreadth distal to the acromion, crossing the humeral head and terminating just above the distal growth plate. Its proximal end must be well anchored in the humeral head, so as not to interfere with shoulder range of motion (Fig. N°59).

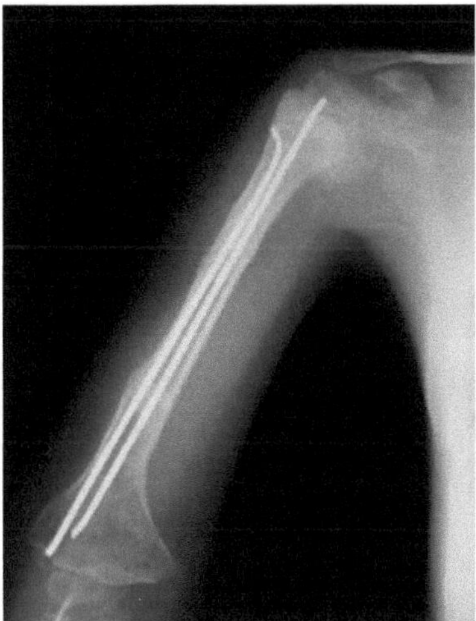

Figure N°59: Radiological image of an ETC of the humerus [personal collection].

Both forearm bones:

Synthesis of the radius is difficult, and the wire has to be bent to try and preserve the radial curvature. The wire is inserted percutaneously from the radial styloid and brought up to the proximal growth plate of the radius. The ulnar wire is lowered from the tip of the olecranon to the distal cartilage of the ulna (Fig. N°60).

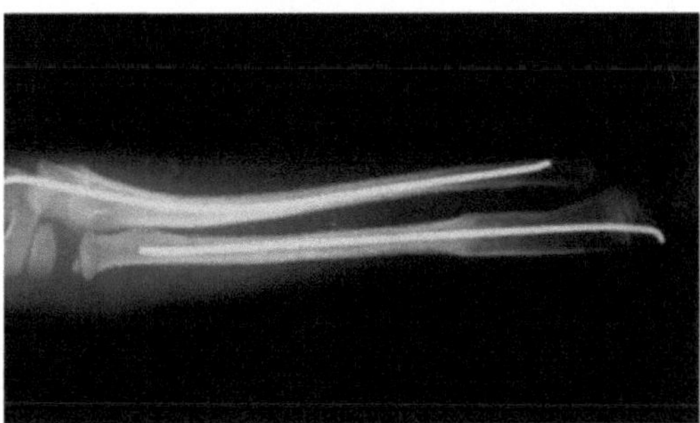

Figure N°60: Radiological image of an ETC of the two bones of the forearm [personal collection].

Femur:

Through a small lateral incision on the knee, a curved pin is pushed through the lateral condyle up to the femoral neck, if possible before the cephalic growth plate. The second is lowered through a small incision opposite the greater trochanter. It penetrates from the trochanter-cephalic junction and descends to the distal cartilage of the femur. Care must be taken to ensure that the femoral neck is in the coxa-valga position (Fig. N°61).

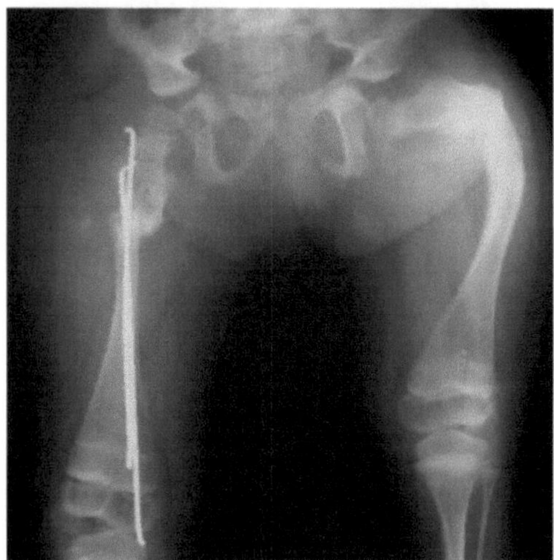

Figure N°61: Radiological image of an ETC of the femur [personal collection].

Leg:

The first pin is inserted from top to bottom, from the prespinal area down to the distal growth plate via a small lateral approach. The second is brought up from the medial malleolar tip to below the proximal cartilage of the tibia (Fig. N°62). These pins are inserted under radiological (scopic) control.

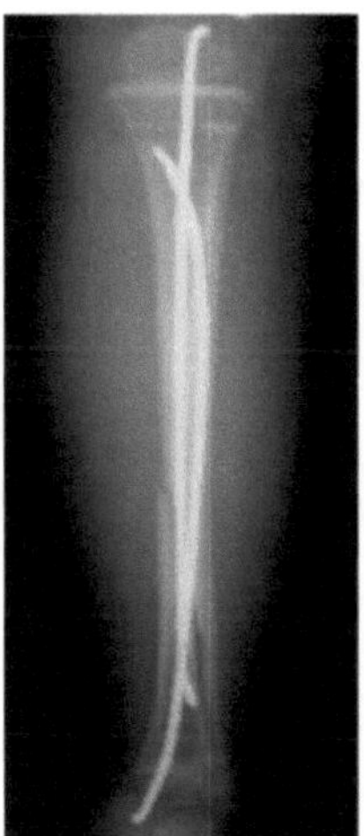

Figure N°62: *Radiological image of ECT of the tibia [personal collection].*

IX.4.2.2. Telescopic subperiosteal sliding pin :

Sub-periosteal pinning (Fig. N°63) is performed after an extensive approach to the bone. The periosteum is incised to expose the diaphysis, alignment is obtained by multiple osteotomies, and then two wires are placed on either side of the corrected diaphysis to secure it. These pins are secured to the bone with a coarse wire hoop. The proximal end of the descending wire is inserted into the proximal epiphysis of the bone, while the distal end of the ascending wire is inserted into the distal epiphysis of the bone. The periosteum is closed over the material. The periosteum will induce ossification that will encompass the fixture. This technique was first described by George Finidori [29].

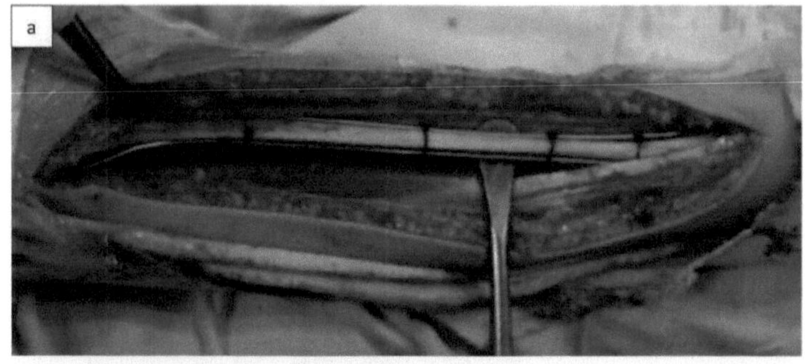

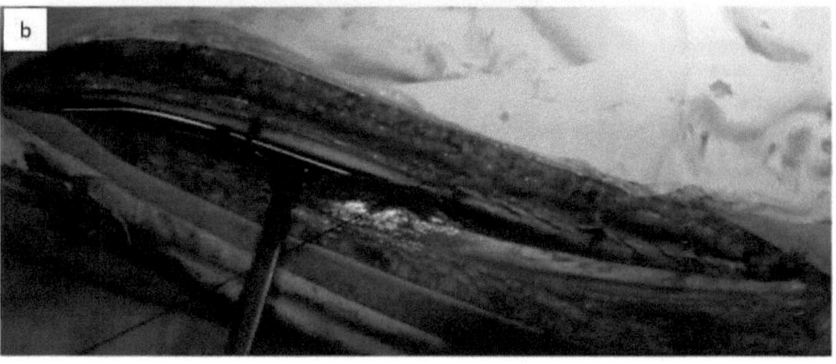

Figure 63: Operative view of subperiosteal telescopic pinning [personal collection] a- Subperiosteal fixation of pins b- Periosteal suture

IX.4.2.3. Mixed telescopic or sliding spindles :

In this variant of telescopic pinning, one pin is inserted into the diaphyseal shaft, while the second, which is impossible to insert into the medullary canal, is placed under the periosteum after de-periostealizing one face of the bone to be treated (Fig. N°64). The periosteum closed over the wire will produce bone. This bone will enclose the wire, which will become intrabony with time.

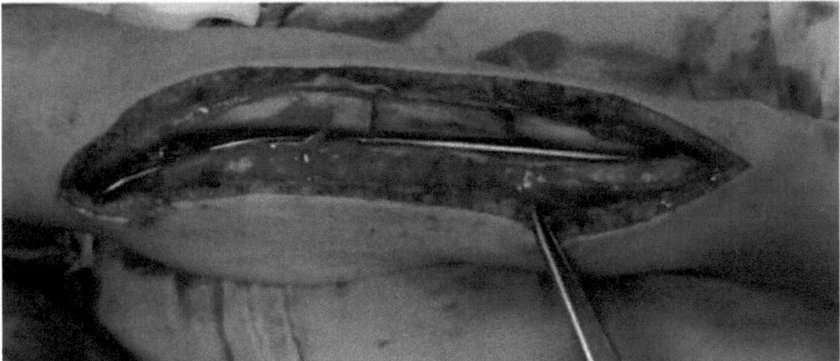

Figure 64: Intraoperative view of mixed pinning [personal collection].

IX.4.3 Preoperative radiological planning :

The following table (Table n°07) summarizes the 6 anatomopathological types, the lesion components of each type and all the surgical procedures required to achieve good bone correction.

TYPE	ANAPATH	PLANIFICATION OPERATOIRE
I	•Pas de déformations •+/- fractures	•Embrochage télescopique intra médullaire (ETIM).
II	•Angle de déformation < 30°. •+/- fractures.	•EIM. •Ostéoclasie. •Ostéotomie percutanée.
III	•Déformation dans 2 plans. •Angle de courbure principal [30°-50°]. •+/- fractures.	•ETIM. •Ostéotomie percutanée. •Ostéotomie a ciel ouvert.
IV	•Déformations sévères dans plusieurs plans. •Angle de déformation principale > 50°. •Fût diaphysaire libre. •+/- fractures.	•ETIM. •Une a plusieurs ostéotomies.
V	•Déformations sévères. •Angle de déformations >50°. •Fût diaphysaire obstrué partiellement. •+/- fractures.	•ETIM, mixte ou sous périostée •Une a plusieurs ostéotomies •Repérméabilisation du fût diaphysaire
VI	•Déformations sévères. •Angle de déformations >50°. •Fût diaphysaire obstrué dans une grande partie. •+/- coxa vara fémorale. •+/- fractures.	•ETIM, mixte ou sous périostée. •Une a plusieurs ostéotomies. •Repérméabilisation du fût diaphysaire. •Correction obligatoire de la coxa vara.

IX.5. Deformation correction :

IX.5.1. Deformity correction and diaphyseal alignment:

Surgical approaches to deformities must be cautious. De-periosteal surgery should be minimal and only necessary. It must be followed by rigorous hemostasis to minimize blood loss. Haemostatic wax can even be used, and some surgeons use an electric scalpel to perform this procedure. At the end of the procedure, the periosteum must be closed to promote consolidation and allow hemostasis by compression [29].

The deformation correction is obtained either :

- By osteoclasia under radiological control when the deformity is minimal and the bone supple.
- Percutaneous osteotomies for minor deformities.
- Open air in large deformations.

The location and number of osteotomies are predefined by preoperative radiological analysis of the deformity and its extent.

Correction osteotomies must comply with classic principles:

- In any case, diaphyseal fragments, especially intermediate ones, should be de-periostealized as little as possible.

- In the case of multiple osteotomies, before performing another osteotomy, it is preferable to ream the intermediate fragment before performing the next osteotomy.
- In flat-bone osteotomies, oblique osteotomies should be preferred, as they offer more bone contact during correction of the deformity, which is conducive to better consolidation [143].
- Osteotomies performed with an oscillating saw should be avoided, as the inter-fragmentary surfaces are burned, which is detrimental to consolidation. Postage stamp osteotomies are preferred [147].
- It is sometimes necessary to perform bone resections to achieve alignment. This resection is best performed with a bone rongeur, while respecting the osteoperiosteal hinge in front of the resection.
- As many diaphyseal osteotomies as necessary can be performed to realign a diaphysis (figure N°65). If the deformity is very severe, bone shortening should not be avoided [143].

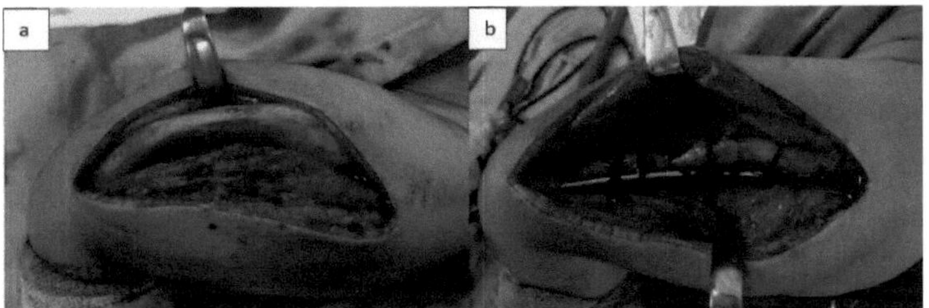

Figure 65: *Multiple osteotomy [personal collection] a- Severe femoral deformity with flat, solid bone b- Multiple osteotomy combined with subperiosteal pinning*

IX.5.2. Correcting basin deformations :

The management of bony manifestations of the pelvis concerns femoral neck fractures, coxa vara and acetabular protrusion.

IX.5.2.1. Fracture of the neck :

It most often occurs on a long varus neck and a mobile hip. It is logical to treat this fracture with an osteosynthesis that allows compression of the fracture and valgization of the neck to reduce the overhang of the upper end of the femur. A combination of localized synthesis of the upper end of the femur to maintain neck valgus and sliding centromedullary osteosynthesis to protect the rest of the femur is often used. Cervico-cephalic epiphysiodesis is preferable. Osteosynthesis without this epiphysiodesis has the disadvantage, in young children, of allowing residual neck growth to develop. As the cervix becomes partially protected, it will varify and eventually fracture [29], [143], (figure N°66).

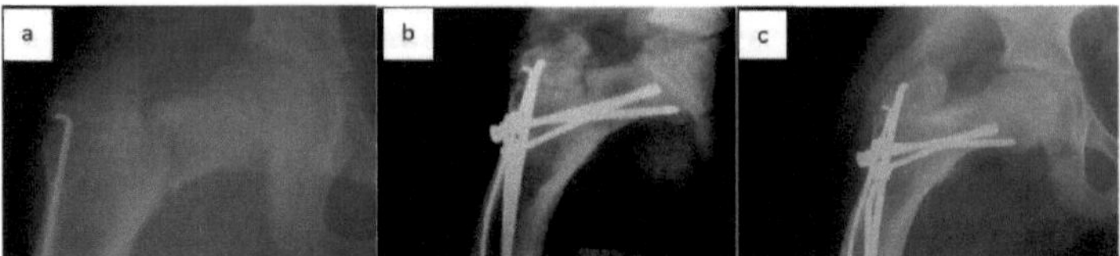

Figure N°66: *Femoral neck fracture and evolution [personal collection]* **I** *a-Radiograph of a femoral neck fracture*
b- Postoperative radiography
c- X-ray at 8-month follow-up

Coxa vara [29], [143], [154] is a very common deformity in osteogenesis imperfecta, often leading to neck fractures. It poses a major problem in the correction of femoral deformities.

It must be prevented whenever femoral alignment is required, taking care to always place the femoral neck in valgus (Figure N°67).

To correct a coxa vara by nailing or pinning, a diaphyseal osteotomy is performed 2 to 3 centimetres below the trochanteric region. The proximal femoral segment is translated medially, bringing the neck into valgus.

The centromedullary material, introduced at the cervical-trochanteric junction, emerges and rests on the lateral cortex of the upper end of the femur, then enters the distal shaft. The apex of the distal femoral fragment rests on the outer surface of the proximal fragment, thus blocking the valgus correction. The neck is thus verticalized [155].

In older children, when the external cortex is fragile, when the varus is cervical or cervico-cephalic, and in severe forms of osteogenesis imperfecta, it is prudent to secure the assembly with a complementary segmental osteosynthesis (screw plate, nail plate or pediatric blade plate) associated with the centromedullary assembly [143].

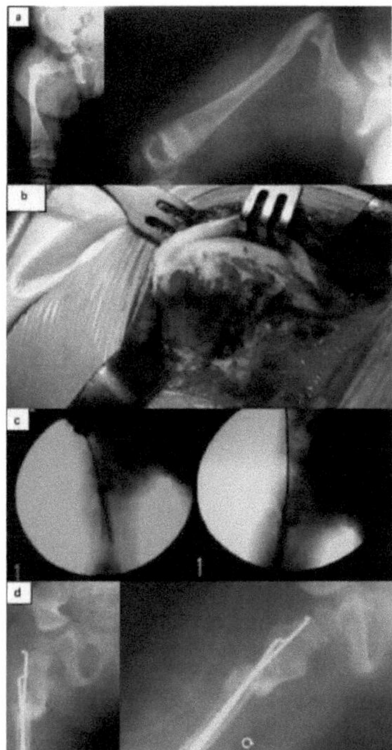

Figure 67: *Correction of an induced coxa vara [personal collection].*
b- Intraoperative view of the deformity of the proximal end of the femur
c- Placement of the fixture under fluoroscopic control d- Front and side x-
rays of the proximal end of the femur after correction

IX.5.2.3. Acetabular protrusion:

In severe forms of osteogenesis imperfecta, the hips are often protruding and not very mobile (figure N°68). The occurrence of a fracture does not necessitate its synthesis. On the contrary, the fracture should be allowed to evolve into a pseudarthrosis of the neck, which becomes providential. This pseudarthrosis will allow a certain degree of hip mobility [143].

In the case of a stiff hip with acetabular protrusion without neck fracture, where intervention on the femur is required, it is important to avoid protecting the neck with osteosynthesis so as not to lose the possibility of a providential pseudarthrosis [143].

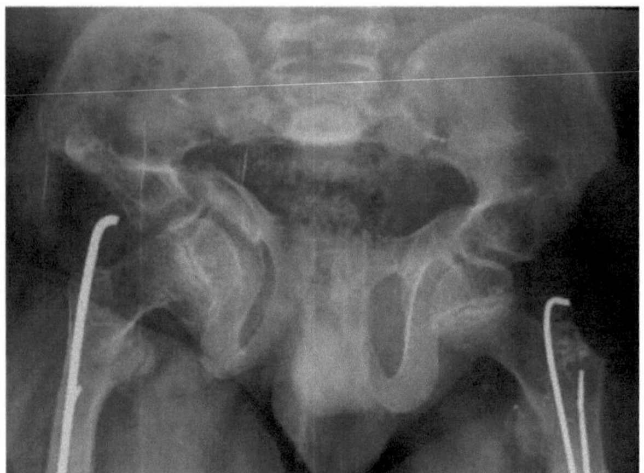

Figure N°68: *Front view of the pelvis showing bilateral acetabular protrusion with deformation of the iliac wings [personal collection].*

IX.6. Related gestures :

IX.6.1. Repermeabilization of the shaft :

Obstruction of the shaft may be :

* Simple and short, the obstacle occupies one or more small areas of the medullary canal.
* Extensive obstruction of a large part of the diaphyseal shaft.
* Total, preventing any permeability of the medullary canal.

Repermeabilization of partially obstructed diaphyseal shafts is carried out by reaming the canal with drill bits of increasing diameter under radiological supervision during preparation of the path for placement of the centromedullary material. In the case of major root canal obstructions, the procedure can be carried out visually, using a back-and-forth technique. This is most often the case when deformities are severe and oriented in several planes of space. This obstruction is secondary to numerous, adjacent fracture calluses (Fig. N°69).

In some cases, the shaft is completely obstructed, and the bone is flat and fragile, with significant deformities. In such cases, canal repermeabilization is impossible, hence the importance of subperiosteal pinning.

If an area of bone located between two osteotomies needs to be repermeabilized, this area should be drilled before the second osteotomy is performed, to avoid de-periostering this intermediate fragment through drilling manoeuvres [147].

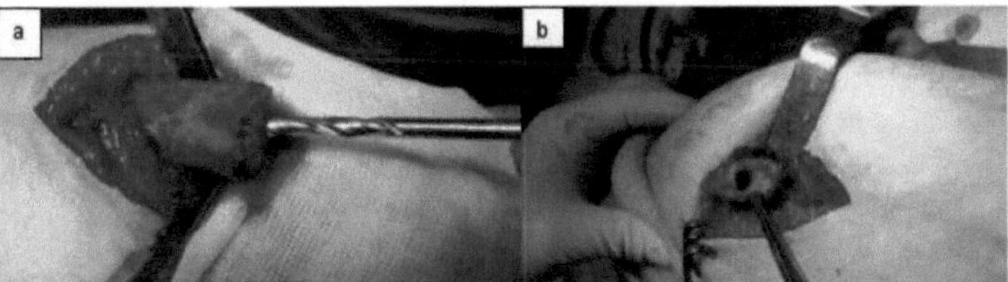

Figure N°69: medullary repermeabilization drilling [personal collection]: a- Manual drilling b- Repermeabilized casing

IX.6.2. Tendon lengthening and aponeurotomy:

In certain forms of severe, inveterate deformity, the muscular course shortens, generating tendinomuscular retractions that sometimes prevent alignment of the long bones. These retractions may persist despite significant bone shortening.

These muscle cords are common:

- Ankle:

Large curvatures of the tibia cause retraction of the posterior muscular loge, which often results in irreducible equinus of the foot, preventing walking. In such cases, percutaneous or de visu (Fig. N°70) tenotomy of the Achilles may be indicated [29], [147].

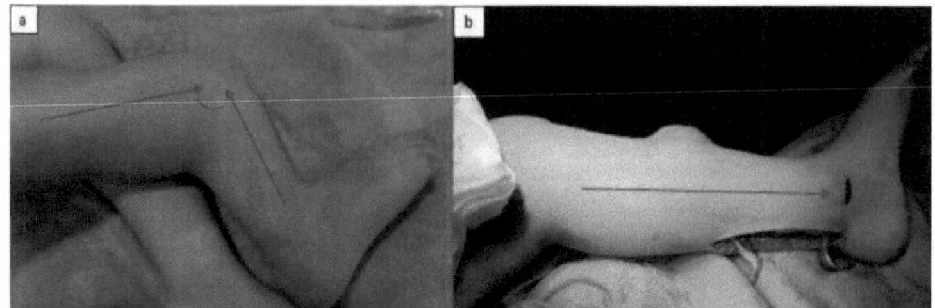

Figure 70: Image of Achilles tendon lengthening [personal collection] a- Angular deformation of the leg b- Leg aligned after Achilles lengthening

- At the hip :

Severe deformities of the femur may cause hip flexion and adductus. This attitude is incompatible with walking, requiring tenotomies of the fascia lata, the direct tendon of the rectus femoris and the tendons of the hip adductor muscles (Figure N°71).

These retractions could lead to femoral neck fractures or aggravate induced coxa vara.

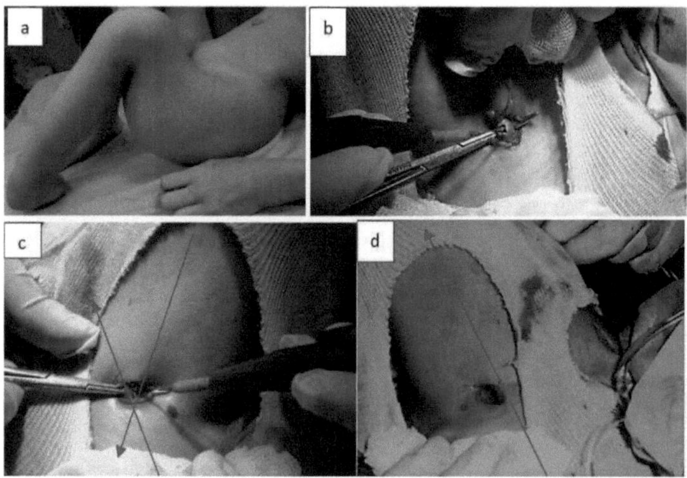

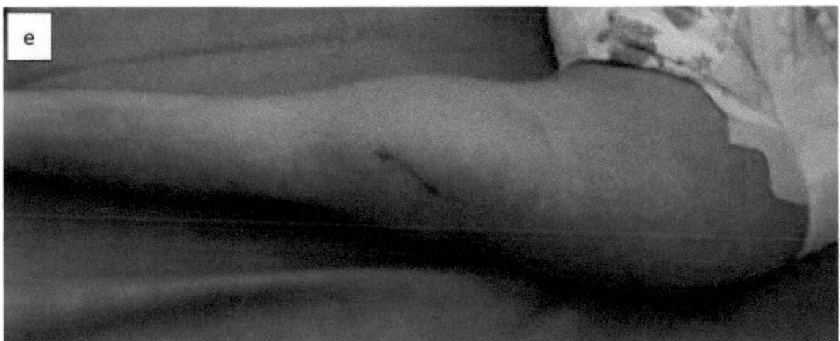

Figure N°71: Peri-articular tenotomies of the hip [personal collection] a- Inveterate deformity of the thigh b- Tenotomy of the adductors c- Tenotomy of the rectus anterior and tensor fascia-lata d- Alignment of the thigh e- Alignment of the thigh at D15 postoperatively

In some cases, in order to combat these retractions and not cause great losses in limb length, it is preferable [143] :

- In the first stage of the operation, osteotomies are performed at the apexes of the deformities, and the limb is then put under short-term stress-relieving traction.
- Secondly, to perform osteosynthesis.

In major corrections using multiple, stepped osteotomies, it is prudent to perform aponevrotomies to avoid the occurrence of compartment syndrome. In the leg, when alignment is achieved by multiple osteotomies, at least the aponevrotomy of the anterolateral compartment should be performed [143].

IX.6.3. Bone graft :

Cortical or cancellous bone grafts are used to treat pseudarthrosis and loss of bone substance.

The cortical graft is cut into flakes on bank bone.

According to the team at Necker Enfants Malades [143], the cortical graft is best incorporated in the femur and less well in the tibia.

In the femur, the graft can be screwed or strapped (Figure N°72).

On the tibia, the graft must be embedded and placed as an inlay by trephining the operated segment (Fig N°72).

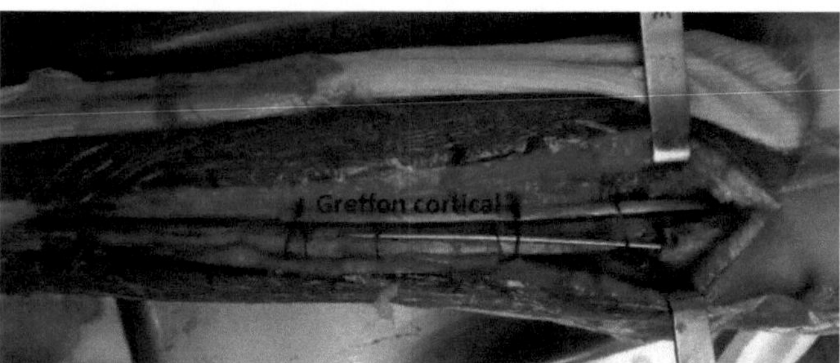

Figure 72: Operative view of a cortical graft on the tibia [collection of G. FINIDORI].

The cancellous graft is divided into small grains, used to boost consolidation and complement a cortical graft.

VARU PUVANESARAJAH et AL [156] have demonstrated the value of sandwiching cortical grafts to treat pseudarthrosis in adults with osteogenesis imperfecta. The allograft is completely integrated into the native bone.

IX.7. Complementary procedures :

IX.7.1 Postoperative immobilization:

Post-operative immobilization can be provided by several methods. It is important to bear in mind the rotation problems that may arise with centromedullary osteosynthesis [143] [147] [148].

- For the lower limbs, this restraint can be provided :
- With a lightweight pedal plaster cast, made either with plaster, conventional resin or, better still, with a lighter flexible resin.
- A long posterior cast splint from the buttock to the foot.
- Pre-molded orthoses postoperatively.
- For the upper limb, immobilization can be provided :
- A posterior splint molded onto the sleeping patient and held in place by an elbow-to-body bandage.
- By a Vietnamese bandage / Gilchrist bandage/ Mayo Clinic
- With a thoraco-brachial orthosis elbow to body: STEVENSON splint
-

The duration of immobilization should be as short as possible, three to four weeks being sufficient. Six weeks should not be exceeded [143] [147] [148].

IX.7.2. Reloading :

For walking children, ambulation must be progressive. It can be done in weightlessness, in the swimming pool, then with a short orthosis until the child is fully supported and walking again.

For non-walking children who are able to walk, the procedure is the same, with long orthoses providing support. Acquisition of walking is slower. Walking is achieved using adapted rehabilitation and learning methods. It is often necessary to use a rocking table to acquire a standing position. Once the child has accepted full weight-bearing, it is time to move on to the use of cuffs, walkers and crutches [157].

IX.7.3. Medical treatment and surgery :

Medical treatment has been implicated in delayed consolidation of fractures and osteotomies in children treated with bisphosphonate.

For LE MERRER and FINIDORI [158], in a series of 27 patients, 30% developed delayed consolidation or pseudarthrosis despite increased bone density. Caution must therefore be exercised, and it is recommended to distance surgery from medical treatment.

Medical treatment has also modified bone consistency, making it more solid. This solidity requires the use of power drills for root canal drilling.

Bisphosphonate overdoses have also been observed, leading to iatrogenic osteopetrosis, sometimes resulting in bone splintering during surgical manipulation.

For FRANÇOIS FASSIER, before the era of bisphosphonates, bone was very fragile to handle and easily crushed. Today, bone is more resistant and osteotomies are more difficult to control, often resulting in splintering [157].

For some authors [149], medical treatment with bisphophonate has no influence on consolidation times.

IX.8. Complications :

IX.8.1. Irradiation and radiology :

For any intramedullary placement, it is essential to have a high-quality preoperative radiological workup. The radiological work-up should include at least front and side views, centered on the plane of the most significant deformity. These images are important for preparing the nailing or pinning material and the intraoperative procedures to be associated with it.

In addition to these important images for the surgeon, these patients are often in possession of a large number of X-rays taken during the diagnostic work-up and during periods of therapeutic follow-up prior to surgery.

All the more so since the procedure is radiosurgical, where radiation spares neither the surgeon nor the patient. It turns out that these children are exposed to a significant and unassessed level of radiation.

Radiology remains the only means of monitoring bone consolidation and assessing the outcome of surgery during growth.

This means that radiology is required before, during and after surgery, throughout the entire follow-up period. This implies that these patients receive a high level of radiation throughout their lives.

These irradiations inflicted on growing children with a long life expectancy will lead to an accumulation of increasing radiation doses, which could have an impact on the patient himself and his offspring [159].

At present, it is certain that repeated radiological surveillance of scoliotic girls and tuberculosis patients is incriminated in the occurrence of cancers, especially breast cancer in women [160], [161], [162].

Overuse of X-rays should be avoided, as there is a risk of radiation-induced cancer. This risk is real for children, given the rapid development and growth of cells, which are more sensitive to radiation [163], [164].

This is why it is so important to justify and optimize examinations using radiation. Recent technical developments in imaging have brought new developments in this direction.

The EOS system (GEORGE CHARPAK, Nobel Prize in Physics 1992), based on digital radiology, allows 2D images to be obtained in a functional position, from head to foot, standing or seated, while reducing the radiation dose thanks to gas sensors (figure N°73).

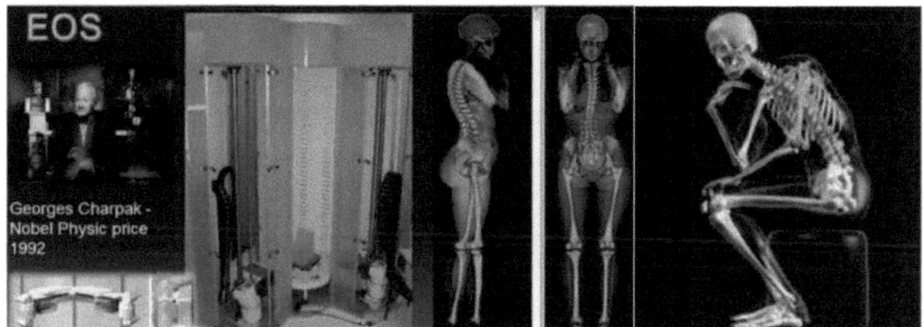

Figure 73: *illustration of the EOS system*

In addition to image quality superior to that of radiographs obtained with standard digital systems, it offers the possibility of 3D reconstruction of all osteoarticular levels. This system enables studies of osteoarticular pathology never before possible [165].

IX.8.2. Cortical resorption :

In osteogenesis imperfecta, the bone is already poorly corticalized. The use of excessively bulky metal hardware leads to bone resorption around the implant. Stainless steel pins 2-2.5mm in diameter are often used in the leg and humerus. Nails of 3.5 to 5 mm are suitable for femurs, and small-diameter KIRCHNER wires are often used for the forearm.

When replacing an osteosynthesis, it is preferable to use a lighter, thinner material. A thinner nail or simple centromedullary pins should be used [143].

IX.8.3. Material fracture :

For some authors, the percentage of fractures in nailing is lower than in pinning [153].

Often, these fractures are of no consequence, as the centromedullary material effectively protects the diaphysis. A short period of immobilization allows the fracture to heal.

Sometimes, the velocity of the trauma causes deformation of the centromedullary material. This deformation must be corrected in the operating room. The material is straightened by external maneuvering under general anesthesia. It is always preferable to keep the original material, especially if it is well fitted and still ensures protection of the entire diaphysis [143].

If it is impossible to straighten the material, or if it no longer protects the bone segment, it must be replaced, in preparation for an often difficult surgical revision [143].

It should be noted that telescopic nails are stiffer than telescopic pins. For identical stresses, there is a risk of more varus deformity occurring in skewered femurs than in nailed femurs [153].

IX.8.4. Hypertrophic callus :

Fractures in osteogenesis imperfecta type V are often complicated by hypertrophic bone callus. Non-steroidal anti-inflammatory treatment postoperatively, or even preventively preoperatively, may be warranted to limit the risk of developing this complication [29], [166].

IX.8.5. Sepsis :

Sepsis is infrequent, the bone is fragile but well vascularized, and patients have no immune deficiency.

In the event of infection, the material should be removed, infected tissue excised, microbiological samples taken and the patient placed on appropriate antibiotic therapy. Once the infection is under control, a new centromedullary osteosynthesis should be performed a few months later [143].

IX.8.6. Hardware migration :

Migration of intraosseous or extraosseous hardware, telescopic nails or telescopic wires appears to be due to poor hardware implantation or the use of inappropriately sized hardware [153], [167].

IX.8.7. Pseudarthrosis :

Pseudarthrosis is common in osteogenesis imperfecta.

It is rare in centromedullary nailing. Reaming the shaft during nail insertion stimulates consolidation.

For BOUTAUD and LAVILLE [153], it is also rare in telescopic pinning. The elasticity of the pins stimulates osteogenesis, because the pins do not absorb all the mechanical stresses in place of the bone. These micromovements are conducive to consolidation [168].

For some authors [158], bisphosphonate treatment has been incriminated as a cause of pseudarthrosis in osteogenesis imperfecta.

POPKOV et al [169] introduced the circular external fixator in the treatment of femoral pseudarthrosis in a child with osteogenesis imperfecta.

IX.8.8. Epiphysiodesis :

Physiological epiphysiodesis is seen mainly in severe forms (popcorn epiphysis). They are due to damage to the growth plate.
Iatrogenic epiphysiodesis is rare. Most often, they are caused by trauma to the growth plate by untimely manoeuvres.
In modern nails, epiphysiodesis is caused by screw insertion of the implant and epiphyseal pull-outs during certain insertion manoeuvres [10].

IX.8.9. Inequality of lower limb length

It may be caused by spontaneous epiphysiodesis of diseased growth plate. In this case, the inequality is minimal.
In severely deformed forms, it is difficult to control limb equalization during surgical correction.
Inequality of length can occur as a result of iatrogenic epiphysiodesis caused by the centromedullary implant during faulty placement.

IX.8.10. Complications specific to telescopic nails :

Telescopic nailing has its own complications. These same complications vary from one type of nail to another. For many authors [150], [170], [171]. These complications range from 33.7% to 72%.
Nail migration with cortical perforation or articular injury appears to be greater in newer nails [170].
T-piece uncoupling is common, especially in the classic BAILLEY and DUBOW nail [11], [172].
Lack of elongation with arrested growth of the child is secondary to a sliding defect of the male part in the female part [170].

IX.9 Indications and surgical strategy:

Not all children with osteogenesis imperfecta require nailing or telescopic pinning.
Telescopic nailing or pinning of the lower limbs is indicated In cases of repeated

fractures or worsening angulation of the limb deformity.

Centromedullary osteosynthesis of the lower limbs is necessary as soon as diaphyseal angulation exceeds 20° [157], or as soon as deformities increase and worsen due to bone loss caused by repeated and prolonged immobilization.

This type of osteosynthesis is also indicated for fractures that occur at the onset of standing and walking [157].

According to GEORGE FINIDORI [143], indications for surgery are rare before the age of 18 months.

In severe and severe forms, simple percutaneous telescopic pinning procedures are recommended, without waiting for major deformations to occur.

For the upper limbs, the indication for osteosynthesis generally comes later. It is indicated when functional difficulties arise, such as the use of crutches, canes or wheelchairs [143], [157].

Repetition of fractures in children, especially those treated with bisphosphonates to improve autonomy after the acquisition of lower-limb corrections. Telescopic nails are frequently used on the humerus and femur.

Telescopic or sliding pinning is preferred for the tibia. This technique presents fewer complications than telescopic nailing.

For both forearm bones, there is no alternative to telescopic sliding pinning. This is the only possible technique for growing children.

The choice of implant is also subject to two criteria [157] :

- Growth: at the end of growth and in the absence of growth potential, as in the case of "popcorn" epiphyses, there is no point in using a sliding system.

- The diameter of the medullary canal: if the medullary canal is too thin and the diaphyseal cortices are thin, reaming the diaphyseal shaft to accommodate a telescopic nail will cause bone loss, and the mechanical stress induced by metal hardware will progressively erode cortical bone reserves. In cases where several bone segments need to be treated and several centromedullary osteosyntheses performed, there is no consensus strategy.

In the lower limb, osteosynthesis of both segments (femur and leg) should be performed in the same operation. Anesthetic risks and hospital stay should be minimized.

It makes more sense to start with the femur first, which will allow the leg to be operated on under a pneumatic tourniquet to minimize blood loss.

On the upper limb, for the same reasons as above, the humerus is operated on first, followed by the two bones of the forearm in the same operating time.

The choice of side is guided by the patient's request, the extent of the deformity and its functional impact.

It is rare to be able to operate on an upper limb and a lower limb at the same time, given the difficulties involved in setting up the patient and the length of the operation.

For some authors [157] and in certain circumstances, it is possible to operate on both upper and lower limbs in the same operative session when the deformities are small and their correction could be performed percutaneously.

X. SURGICAL TREATMENT OF SPINAL DEFORMITIES:

Spinal deformities complicate the functional and vital prognosis in osteogenesis imperfecta, especially in severe forms [173], [174], [175].

Vertebral fractures, platispondylia, spinal growth disorders, muscular deficits, particularly of the respiratory muscles, and hyperlaxity are responsible for thoraco-rachidic manifestations [175].

Static disorders of the spine are complex, often associating scoliosis, dorsolumbar kyphosis and dorsal lordosis. These disorders act in all three planes of space, adding to the patient's short stature and trunk deformity [82], [175].

In addition to the mechanical repercussions, these spinal disorders aggravate the patient's functional state through pain phenomena, splanchnomegaly secondary to elevations of the diaphragmatic cupolas and respiratory failure due to restriction of the pulmonary fields [175].

This respiratory failure is the main cause of mortality in osteogenesis imperfecta.

At the cervico-cephalic hinge, basilar protrusion (Figure 74) is not uncommon. This situation can lead to spinal cord compression, hydrodynamic disorders of the cerebrospinal fluid (CSF) and the formation of syringomyelia. [82], [175].

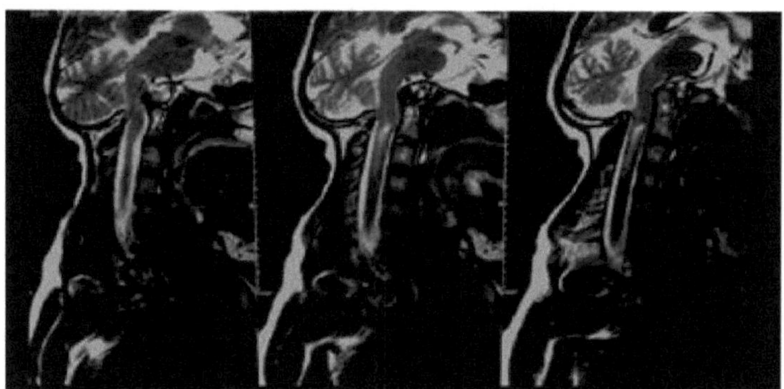

Figure N°74: MRI image of basilar protrusion [collection G. Finidori].

Management of respiratory disorders is essential. General rehabilitation, and in particular respiratory rehabilitation, is a priority. It must begin at birth and

114

continue without interruption.

Medical treatment with bisphosphonates has been shown to be effective in treating platispondylia and spinal pain.

Prevention in early childhood plays a major role in the prevention of thoraco-spinal deformities. Some of these measures can be taken by parents right from birth, such as keeping the baby supine, in a straight position, wedged upright with fabric wedges, and giving preference to transporting horizontal babies in strollers and baby carriages.

Orthopedic treatment with corsets is of little or no benefit, especially in severe forms. It reduces patient autonomy, aggravates motor difficulties, limits mobility, increases bone loss, does not prevent worsening of spinal deformities and impairs respiratory function [174], [175].

Surgical treatment with instrumented posterior arthrodesis remains the method of choice in the management of these deformities.

Age and bone maturation are not the only criteria for spinal arthrodesis. In osteogenesis imperfecta, [173], [174], [175] must be taken into account:

- Loss of the patient's sitting height during growth.
- Absence or stoppage of trunk growth.
- Progressive worsening of deformities.
- Loss of reducibility, especially in kyphosis.
- The absence of progression of vital capacity or its decrease (vital capacity < 60%) and the onset of signs of respiratory insufficiency (sleep-disordered breathing).
- Worsening respiratory function impairment and recurrent, severe bronchopulmonary infections.

In osteogenesis imperfecta, it is not necessary to wait until the end of growth to decide whether or not to operate.

Preparation for spinal surgery in osteogenesis imperfecta does not differ greatly from conventional spinal surgery. It requires an obligatory check-up, decided in collaboration between the surgeon and the anesthesiologist [175].

It essentially comprises a clinical, biological and neurological examination, a radiological assessment with front and side spine telemetry, magnetic resonance imaging (MRI) and a spinal CT scan to study vertebral morphology.

Cardiac status is often normal, but respiratory function poses major problems specific to this type of surgery.

For each patient to be operated on:
- Respiratory function must be assessed by means of a respiratory function test (RFT) and plysomnography.

If vital capacity is impaired, special preparation is required. If this capacity is less than one liter, a tracheotomy may be necessary.
- Basilar impression with risk of neuraxial compression associated with syringomyelia must be ruled out. This situation justifies craniotomy, decompression laminectomy and occiputo-cervical arthrodesis.

Preparing the patient by traction with a cranial halo reduces spinal deformity and improves trunk balance [173] (figure N°75).

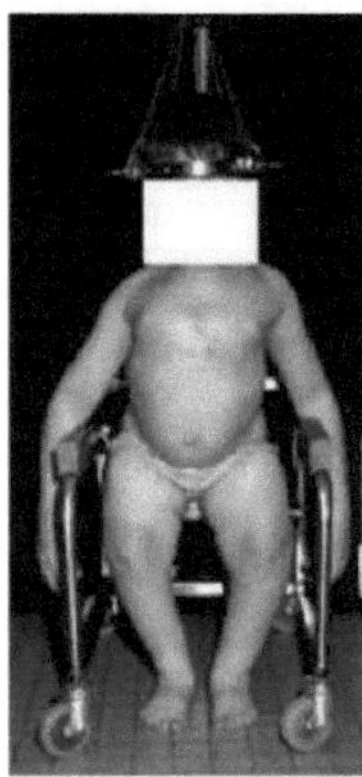

Figure 75: *Chair traction with cranial halo [collection G. FINIDORI].*

This traction is justified in large kyphotic deformities, trunk imbalances and short thoraxes.

Traction is performed in the operating theatre, under general anaesthetic. There should be as many cranial fixation points as possible, generally 8 to 10, distributed around the skull, sparing the frontal and occipital regions.

Traction is applied immediately on awakening, and the weight of the traction is rapidly increased to 30-40% of body weight. It is maintained for 45 to 60 days, with daily neurological monitoring and local care of the fixation points. The effectiveness of traction is regularly assessed by the gain in trunk size and vital capacity, which averages 10 to 30%.

At the end of traction, a repeat radiological assessment of the entire spine and of the spine under traction is required. A follow-up CT scan of the spine is often requested.

In addition to traction, it is sometimes necessary to create an anterior plaster cast in which the patient is operated on in the prone position.

Posterior arthrodesis is the technique of choice for the treatment of vertebral deformities in osteogenesis imperfecta [175].

It is performed in the operating room, with the patient lying prone. In severe cases, the patient is placed on a pre-prepared anterior shell.

Surgery is performed under neurological supervision, using evoked potentials. The patient is kept under traction during the operation, the force of which is reduced to half that used preoperatively.

The spine is approached progressively with an electric scalpel to ensure continuous hemostasis. Blood loss must be minimized and bleeding controlled with appropriate anesthesia.

In reinforced posterior spinal arthrodesis, there is no need to seek an improvement in the correction obtained by preoperative traction; fixation is performed in situ [175].

Posterior vertebral arthrodesis is usually extensive, extending from the first dorsal vertebra to the sacrum, especially in severe forms [175].

This arthrodesis is armed, and osteosynthesis material must be used. Without this, arthrodesis alone cannot protect the spine from the risk of progressive collapse and worsening of deformities [175].

Posterior vertebral arthrodesis is performed using a suitable pediatric titanium vertebral osteosynthesis device combined with an allograft harvested from a bank head mixed with bone fragments obtained during avulsion. Isolated autografting is insufficient.

For GEORGE FINIDORI et al [175], posterior arthrodesis allows :

- Good stabilization of the deformity and correction in 37% of cases.
- Improved respiratory function.
- Greater freedom of movement.
- An average gain in trunk size of 6 cm.
- A zero mortality rate.

Post-operatively, especially in severe forms, endotracheal intubation via the nasal passage should generally be maintained, and respiratory support provided until the patient has recovered effective respiratory function [175].

It would seem preferable to maintain immobilization with a bivalve corset for three to four months.

Sitting is contraindicated for three months in fragile children after correction of large deformities [175].

These surgical patients require effective, long-term respiratory physiotherapy combined with a rehabilitation program in specialized centers to regain maximum autonomy [175].

Correction of these spinal deformities (Fig. N°76) in osteogenesis imperfecta is difficult, but it has been confirmed that this surgery improves patients' functional status. Posterior vertebral arthrodesis appears to preserve vital function and reduce the extent of vertebral and thoracic deformities [82], [175]. As illustrated in the following case :

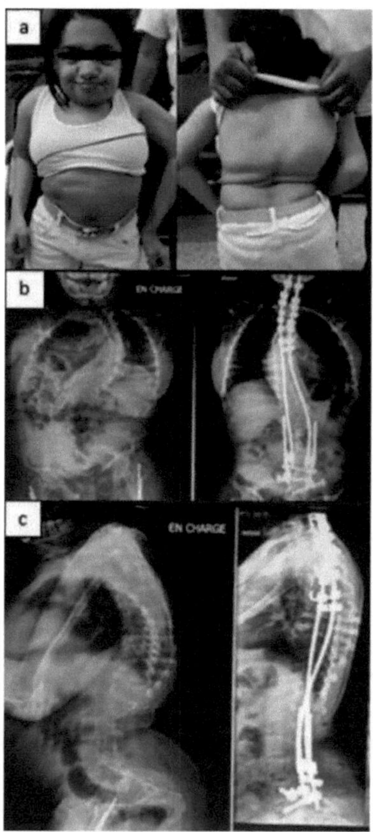

Figure N°76: *Correction of kyphoscoliosis [collection M. Ait Ouarab and K. Hachelaf].*
a- Clinical appearance of kyphoscoliosis

b- Front radiograph of the spine before and after correction
c- Spine X-ray before and after profile correction

XI. CONCLUSION

Osteogenesis imperfecta is a rare pathology characterized by bone fragility. It is genetic in origin, autosomal dominant in 90% of cases and recessive in the remaining 10%. It mainly affects collagen production.

This genetic defect is responsible for bone and extra-bone manifestations of variable expression.

Its management has been a long road, from the identification and classification of this pathology, to medical treatment and finally surgical management.

Molecular biology research and the identification of the genomes responsible for this condition have made it possible to develop and guide targeted medical therapy.

Surgical treatment is an important piece of the puzzle in the palliative management of this mysterious disease.

The wealth of literature published in recent years demonstrates the interest of medical research in this pathology.

Surgery has moved on from the era of bone fragmentation, allowing alignment of the diaphyses and restraint with a single SOFIELD nail, to the minimally invasive techniques with restraint with a telescopic BAILLEY and DUBOW nail [11] developed by FASSIER and DUVAL [10] and others.

Telescopic pinning, introduced in 1987 by METAIZEAU [12], is part of the arsenal of osteosynthesis techniques used in surgery for osteogenesis imperfecta. The principles of wire insertion were further developed by GEORGE FINIDORI [29]. The particularities of this technique have enabled it to carve out an important place for itself among the modern means used in this type of surgery.

The success of any surgical procedure depends not only on technical mastery, but also on multidisciplinary management involving pediatricians, rheumatologists, rehabilitation specialists, physiotherapists, psychologists, patients' parents and society as a whole.

APPENDICES

Appendix 1: List of figures

Appendix 2: List of tables

References

1. [List of rare diseases as well as pharmaceutical products intended for their treatment. Journal Officiel de la République Algérienne N°50 du 03 Octobre 2013].

2. [chevrel, guillaume. Ostéogenèse imparfaite de l'adulte, etude absorpleometrie et therapeutique Th: Med: Lyon I: 1996, 1-40].

3. [Kreps-Sellam Monique, Kreps François. Osteogenesis imperfecta through history... in a few dates. L'ostéogenèse imparfaite: Maladie des os de verre/Pierre Verhaeghe. 2nd edition. Paris: Frisson Roche, 1999, P. 18-19].

4. [Eve J. Lowenstein Osteogenesis imperfecta in a 3,000-year-old mummy. Childs Nerv Syst (2009) 25:515-516. Osteogenesis imperfecta 10.1007/s00381-009-0817-7].

5. [Aufderheide AC, Rodriguez-Martin C (1998) The Cambridge. encyclopedia of human paleopathology. Cambridge University. Press, Cambridge].

6. [Delhi N. Reminiscences from Indian Pediatrics: A Tale of 50 Years Tubercular Meningitis A Tale of 50 Years 2016. doi: 10. 3389/fmicb. 2015.00791].

7. [Louis V., Avioli Stephen M., krane. Metabolic bone disease and clinically related disorders. Third Edition, 1998: 651-52].

8. [DevoglaerJp, Malghem J, Maldagne B, Nagant de Deuxchaine C. Radiological manifestations of panidronate in children with severe osteogenesisimperfecta. Med 1998; 339: 947-52].

9. [Sofield HA and Miller EA. Fragmentation, realignment and intramedullary rod Fixation of the deformety of the long bone of children. A ten-year approval. J Bone Joint Surg; 42-A: 1371; 1959].

10. [Fassier F and Al. Multicenter Radiological assessment of the Fassier-Duval femoral rodding, POSNA, San Diego 2006]

11. [Bailey RW, Dubow HI. Study of longitudinal bone growth resulting in an extensible nail. Surg Forum 1963; 14 :455-458]

12. [Metaizeau JP. Sliding centro-medullary nailling. Application to the treatment of severe forms of osteogenesis imperfecta. Chir Pediatr. 1987; 28(4-5): 240-243]

13. [Weil UH .Osteogenesis imperfecta: historical background Clin Orthop Relat Res., 1981; 159: 6-10].

14. [P.J. Roughley*, F. Rauch and F.H. Glorieu. Osteogenesis Imperfecta - clinical and molecular diversity Genetics Unit, Shriners Hospital for Children, Montreal, Canada, European Cells and Materials Vol. 5. 2003 (Pages 41-47) Dostéogenèse imperfecta: 10.2].

15. [F. Fassier, F.H. Glorieux. Osteogenesis imperfecta in children. SOFCOT 1999; 70: 235-252].

16. [Koche rand Shaprio. Osteogenesis imperfecta. J of American Academy of Orthop Surg. 6 (4): 225- 360. July 1998]

17. [D. Primorac, JW. Rowe, M. Mottes, I. Barisic, D. Anlicevic, S. Mirandola, F. Glorieux. Osteogenesis imperfecta at the beginning of bone and Joint decade. Croatian Medical Journ. 42(4) 394-415. 2001].

18. [Forin V, osteogenesis imperfecta. Orphanet Encyclopedia. June 2007].

19. [Andersen PE, Jr. and Hauge M. Osteogenesis imperfecta: a genetic, radiological, and epidemiological study. Clin Genet. 1989 Oct; 36(4):250-5. PubMed PMID: 2805382].

20. [Abrahamsen (B), Langdahl (BL), Gram (J) and Brixen (K). Mortality and Morbidity in Patients with Osteogenesis Imperfecta in Denmark. DANISH MEDICAL JOURNAL: 2018; 65(4):B5454].

21. [Forlino A, Marini JC. Osteogenesis imperfecta. Lancet. 2016 Apr 16; 387(10028):1657-71. PubMed PMID: 26542481].

22. [Kuurila K, Kaitila I, Johansson R, Grenman R. Hearing loss in Finnish adults with osteogenesis imperfecta: a nationwide survey. Ann Otol Rhinol Laryngol. 2002 Oct; 111(10):939-46. PubMed PMID: 12389865].

23. [B. Aubry-Rozier, S.Unger, A. Bregou, M. Freymond, Morisod, A. Vaswani, P. Schneider, L. Bonafé. New developments in osteogenesis imperfecta: from research to multidisciplinary management. Rev Med Suisse 2015; 11: 657-62].

24. [Rohrbach M, Giunta C. Recessive osteogenesis imperfecta: Clinical, radiological, and molecular findings. Am J Med Genet C Semin Med Genet 2012; 160C: 175-89].

25. [Van Dijk FS, Zillikens MC, Micha D, et al. PLS3 mutations in X-linked osteoporosis with fractures. N Engl J Med 2013; 369:1529-36].

26. [Rauch F., Travers R., Parfitt AM., Glorieux FH. Static and dynamic bone histomorphometry in children with osteogenesisimperfecta, 2000: 581-89].

27. [Bonafe L, Hasler C, Janner M, et al. Osteogenesis imperfecta: clinical manifestations, diagnosis and management from childhood to adulthood. Forum Med Suisse2013; 13: 925-31].

28. [Z.Pejin, G.Finidori. Osteogenesis imperfecta. Hôpital des Enfants-Malades. Université René Descartes; 2015].

29. [Finidori G, Toupouchian V, Palliative osteosynthesis in children with osteogenesis imperfecta. La Gazette de la société française d'orthopédie pédiatrique 2007; 22: 24-9].

30. [A. Demeglio, growth in orthopedics. Sauramps médical, 2nd edition. 1991, P22] [J.-L. Jouve, J.-M Guiaume, F. Launay, P.Frayssinet, M. Panuel, G. Bollini. Trauma to the growth plate. Fracture de l'enfant. Monographie du GEOP. Sauramps médical, 2002. P 19-20].

31. [J.-L. Jouve, J.-M Guiaume, F. Launay, P.Frayssinet, M. Panuel, G. Bollini. Trauma to the growth plate. Fracture de l'enfant. Monographie du GEOP. Sauramps médical, 2002. P 19-20].

32. [In Green, Children's Fractures, Saunders 1996].

33. [CHUNG S, BATTERMAN J, BRIGHTON G Schear strength of the human femoral capital epiphyseal plate. J Bone Joint Surg Am, 1976, 58: 94-103].

34. [DE PARLOS J, ALFARO ARIAN C. fractures of the growth plat. In De Plablos, surgery of the growth plate, Madrid, Ediciones Ergon, 1998, 143-170].

35. [Téot L. Stable elastic centromedullary nailing in children. In: Cahiers d'enseignement de la SOFCOT. N°28. Teaching conference. Paris : expansion scientifique ; 1987. P. 71-90].

36. [Kwong NK, Harris MB. Recent developments in the biology of fracture repair. J Am Acad Orthop Surg 2008; 16: 619-25].

37. [Giannoudis PV, Eihorn TA, Schmiedmaier G, Marsh D. the diamond concept-open question. Injury 2008: 39S2: S5-8].

38. [Jepsen K, Price C, Silkman L, et al. Genetic variation in the paterns of sk el et al progenitor cell differentiation and progression during endochondral bone formation affects the rat of fracture healing. J Bone Miner Res 2008; 23: 1204-16].

39. [Horwltz EM, Gordon PL, Koo WKK. Isolated allogenic bone marrow-derived mesenchymal cells engraft and stimulate growth in children with osteogenesin imperfecta: implecation for cell therapy of bone. www. Pnas.org/cgi/doi/10.1073/pnas/132252399].

40. [B de Billy. Osteosynthesis in child and adolescent orthopedics and traumatology. Teaching conference; 2013. Elsevier Masson SAS; p: 183-195].

41. [Meunier P., and P chavassieux. Histology and cytology of normal bone. Encyclopédie Médico-Chirurgicale 14- 002-A-10-2000].

42. [Nguyen S.H. Bone. Manual of anatomy and cytology. 3rd edition. Paris. Lamarre: 2005]

43. [Rossert J., De Gromburgghe B. Type I collagen: structure,synthesis and regulation. In: Bilezikan JP, Raisz LG, Rodan GA eds. Principales of bone biology. San Diego: Academic Press, 1996: 127-42].

44. [Buckwalter JA, Glimcher MJ, Cooper RR, Recker R. Bone biology. Part II: formation, from, modeling, remodeling and regulation of cell function. J Bone It Surg 1995; 77A: 1267-89].

45. [Parfitt AM. Integration of skeletal and mineral homeostasis. In: Deluca HF, Frost H, Jee W, JohnstonC, Parfitt AM eds. Osteoporosis: recent advances in pathogenesis and treatment. University Park, 1981: 115-26].

46. [Agathe OGIER, épouse ECHARD. Multiscale characterization of bone tissue. Application to osteogenesis imperfecta. PhD thesis from the University of Lyon. 21/11/2017].

47. [Bullough P.G., Davdson D.D., Lorenzo J.C. The morbid anatomy of the skeleton in osteogenesis imperfect. Clin. Orthop. 1981, 159, 42-57].

48. [Falvo K.A., Bullough P.G. Osteogenesis imperfecta: a histometric analysis. J. med. Joint. Surg. (AM), 1973; 55-A: 1415-25].

49. [Glorieux F. Bone 2000 - Moira S. Rev Endocr Metab Disord 2008].

50. [Frank Rauch, Francis H Glorieux. Osteogenesis imperfecta ,Seminar 2004.The Lancet].

51. [x. kassa-1 k. hachelaf-2. 1 : anatomopathology department, 2 : orthopedic surgery "B" CHU DOERA]

52. [Sillence D.O., Senn A., Danks D.M. Genetic Heterogeneity in Osteogenesis Imperfecta. J.Med. GENET., 1979; 16: 101-16].

53. [Smith R. Osteogenesis imperfecta. Clinics in Rheumatic Disease, 1986; 12: 655-89].

54. [Chan C.C., Green R., De la cruz Z.C., Hillis A. Ocular findings in ostegenesis imperfecta congenita. Arch Ophthalmol. 1982; 100: 1459-63].

55. [Sharpiro J.R., Pikus A., Weiss G., Rowe D.W. Hearing and middle ear function in ostegenesis imperfecta. Jama. 1982 Apr 16; 247(15): 2120-6].

56. [Delhi N. Reminiscences from Indian Pediatrics: A Tale of 50 Years Tubercular Meningitis. A Tale of 50 Years 2016. doi:10.3389/fmicb.2015.00791].

57. [Louis V., Avioli Stephen M., krane. Metabolic bone disease and clinically related disorders. Third Edition, 1998: 651-52].

58. [Weil UH .Osteogenesis imperfecta: historical background Clin Orthop Relat Res., 1981; 159: 6-10].

59. [Van Dijk FS, Sillence DO. Osteogenesis imperfecta: Clinical diagnosis, nomenclature and severity assessment. Am J Med Genet Part A 2014; 164A:1470-813].

60. [Sillence DO, Rimoin DL. Classification of osteogenesis imperfect. Lancet 1978; 1: 1041-2].

61. [Byes PH. Osteogenesis Imperfecta: perspectives and opportunities. CurrOpin Pediat.2000; 12:603-9].

62. [Sillence DO. Osteogenesis Imperfecta: an expanding of variant. ClinOrthp 1981; 12:603-9].

63. [G. Baujat, C. Michot, G. Pinto, S. Monnot, V. Cormier-Daire. Osteogenesis imperfecta, genetic aspects, medical management. La Gazette de la Société Française d'Orthopédie Pédiatrique. October-November 2016; Num 46; P 2-4].

64. [Marini JC, Reich A, Smith SM. Osteogenesis imperfecta due to mutations in non-collagenous genes: Lessons in the biology of bone formation. Curr Opin Pediatr, 2014; 26: 500-7].

65. [Hoyer-Kuhn H, Netzer C, Koerber F, Schoenau E, Semler O. Two years inverted question mark experience with denosumab for children with steogenesis imperfecta type VI. Orphanet J Rare Dis 2014; 9:145].

66. [Baalbaky I, Manouvrier S, Dufour Ph, Devismes L, Delzenne A, Boute O, Puech F. Antenatal diagnosis of osteogenesis imperfecta. J Gynecol Obstet Biol Reprod. 1998; 27: 44-51].

67. [Zionts LE, Nash JP, Rude R, Ross T, Stott S - Bonne mineral density in children with midl osteogenesis imperfecta. J Bone Joint Surg, 1995; 77B: 143-7].

68. [Véronique FORIN. Osteogenesis imperfecta in children, 2016 update, JPP Paris 2016].

69. [Pierre Verhaeghe, Blandine Gosset. Osteogenesis imperfecta: current situation in children and adults. XVéme journée scientifique du groupe de recherche et d'information sur l'ostéoporose - Paris January 11, 2002].

70. [Glorieux FH, Pettfor JM, Jupner H, editors. Pediatric Bone: Biology and Diseases. San Diego: academic Press; 2003. p. 513-516].

71. [Gamble JG, Rinsky LA, Strudwick J, Bleck EE- non-union of fractures in children who have osteogenesis imperfecta. J Bone Joint Surg, 1988; 70A: 439-43].

72. [Scott NS, Zionts LE - Displaced fractures of the apophysis of olecranon in children who have osteogenesis imperfecta. J Bone Join Surg, 1993; 75A: 1026-33].

73. [Azrak S., Ksyar R., Ben Raïs N. Complications -orthopediques-de-l'osteogenese- imp,em-consulte.com/article/236704/ Médecine Nucléaire 33 (2009) 749-753].

74. [Moorefield WG Jr, Miller GR. Aftermath of osteogenesis imperfecta: the disease in adulthood.J Bone Joint Surg Am. 1980 Jan; 62(1):113-9].

75. Justin Easow Sam, Mala Dharmalingam. Osteogenesis imperfect. Indiana Journal of Endocrinology and Metabolism. Volume 21, Issue 6, p: 903-908. November- December 2017

76. [Trehan SK, Morakis E, Raggio CL, Twomey KD, Green DW. Acetabular Protrusio and Proximal Femur Fractures in Patients With Osteogenesis Imperfecta. J Pediatr Orthop. 2015 Sep;35(6):645-9].

77. [George Finidorie, Paris Necker enfants Malades. The hip in adult osteogenesis imperfecta, Osteogenesis Imperfecta: What happens after childhood? Devenir à l'âge adulte, 8eme Journée de Formation, Friday April 2, 2004 in PARIS (20e)].

78. [Butani L, Rosekrans JA, Morgenstern BZ, Milliner DS- An unusual renal complicationin a patient with osteogenesis imperfecta. Am J Kidney Dis, 1995; 25: 489-91].

79. [Lee JH, Gambel JG, Moore RE, Rinsky LA- Gastrointestinal problems in patients who have type III osteogenesis imperfecta. J Bone Loint Surgy, 1995; 77A: 1352-6].

80. [Rothschild, Leelach, Goeller, Jessica, Voronov, Polina, Barabanova, Alexandra, Smith, Peter. Anesthesia in children with osteogenesis imperfecta: Retrospective chart review of 83 patients and 205 anesthetics over 7 years. Wiley-Blackwell Journals, Pediatric Anesthesia. 2018; Volume2 Question11 Pages1050-1058].

81. [G. Finidori, V Topouchian, Z, Pejin, C Glorion. Surgical treatment of spinal deformities of osteogenesis imperfecta. La Gazette de la Société Française d'Orthopédie Pédiatrique. N°46. October - November 2016. P : 14-18]

82. [Maegen J. Wallace, MD Richard W. Kruse, DO, MBA, Suken A. Shah, MD. The Spine in Patients With Osteogenesis Imperfecta. J Am Acad Orthop Surg 2017;25: 100-109]

83. [V. Forin. Osteogenesis imperfecta in Pathologie phosphocalcique et osseuse de l'enfant - Progrès en pédiatrie. 2015 - Ed Dostéogenèse imparfaiteN], [F. Fassier, F.H. Glorieux. Osteogenesis imperfecta in children. SOFCOT 1999; 70: 235-252].

84. [Marjorana et al. Dentinogenesis imperfecta in children with osteogenesis imperfecta: a clinical and ultrastructural study. International journal of pediatic dentistry. 2010 : 20 ; 212-218].

85. [Malmgren B, Norgren S, Dental aberration in children and adolescents with osteogenesis imperfecta. 2002; 60: 65-71].

86. [Breslau-Siederius LJ, Engelgert RH, Pals G, Van der Sluijs JA - Bruck syndrome: a rare combination of bone fragility and multiple congenital joint contractures. J Pediatr Orthop, 1998; 7B: 35-8].

87. [Mc Pherson E, Clemens M - Burck syndrome (osteogenesis imperfecta with congenital joint contractures): review and report on the first North American case. Am J Med Genet, 1997; 70: 28-31].

88. [Cropp GJA, Myers DN, Physiological evidence of hypermetabolism in osteogenesis imperfect. Pediatrics, 1972; 49: 375-91].

89. [Poesborg P, Astrup D, Lund AM, Ording H. Osteogenesis imperfecta and malignant Hyperthermia. Is there a relationship? Anesthesia. 1996; 51 :863-5].

90. [Remy Nottin. Osteogenesis imperfecta, the future of the heart. Journal de l'association de l'ostéogenèse imparfaite. Paris ; 02 avril 2004].

91. [Wong RS, Follis FM, Shively BK, Wernly JA. Osteogenesis imperfecta and cardiovascular diseases. Ann Thorac Surgy. 1995; 60: 1439-43].

92. [Favier R, Bronstein C, Forin V. Coagulation screening test in 35 children with osteogenesis imperfecta. 8th international conference on osteogenesis imperfect. Annecy 1-3 september 2002].

93. [MC Allcon, J Paterson. Cause of death in osteogenesis imperfect. J Clin Pathol ; 1996, 49 (8) :627- 30].

94. [Véronique FORIN. Osteogenesis imperfecta = glass bone disease = Lobstein's disease = osteogenesis imperfecta. Enseignement National DES - DIU de Médecine Physique et de réadaptation. Module: Physical and rehabilitation medicine in pediatric pathology. St Maurice - February 29, 2012].

95. [Young-Hing K, McEwen GD: Scoliosis associated with osteogenesis imperfecta. J Bone Joint Surg (Br), 1982, 64, 36-43].

96. [Kuurila K, Grenman R. Response to "Is it necessary to screen for hearing loss in the Pediatric population with osteogenesis imperfecta?". clin Otolaryngol Allied Sci. 2004; 29:28. 7].

97. [Kuurila-Svahn K, 10th international conference on osteogenesis imperfecta. Ghent, October 2008].

98. [P. Dupuy. Osteogenesis imperfecta and skin. Osteogenesis imperfecta: glass bone disease/Pierre Verhaeghe. 2nd edition. Paris. Frison Roche, 1999, P 162-165].

99. [Sawin PD, Menezes AH. Basilar invagination in osteogenesis imperfecta and related osteochondrodysplasia: medical and surgical management. J Neurosurg. 1997; 86: 950-60].

100.   [Chamas LR, Marini JC, communicating hydrocephalius, basilar

invagination and other neurologic features in osteogenesis imperfecta.
Neurology, 1993; 43: 2603-8].

101.   [Chines A, Petersen DJ, Schranck FW, Whyte MP. Hypercalciuria in
children severely affected with osteogenesis imperfecta. J Pediatr. 1991; 119: 51-
7].

102.   [Cole DEC-Psychosocial aspect of osteogenesis imperfecta. An Updat. Am
J Med Genet, 1993; 45:207-11].

103.   Looser in 1906

104.   [P. Maroteau. Osteochondrodysplasia. Les maladies osseuses de l'enfant.
3rd edition, 1995. P 165-176].

105.   [Antonella Forlino, Wayne A. Cabral, Aileen M. Barnes and Joan C. Marini:
New perspectives on osteogenesis imperfecta. Nature Review Endocrinolog. Sep
2011; 7, 540-557].

106.   [Snoecky A., Vanhoenacker FM., Parizel PM (2008). Popcorn calcifications
in osteogenesis imperfecta. JBR-BTR, 91:176].

107.   [Obafemi AA., Bulas DI., Troendle J., Marini JC. Popcorn calcification in
osteogenesis imperfecta: incidence, progression, and molecular correlation. Am J
Med Genet A., 2008; 146A: 2725-2732. doi: 10.1002 / ajmg.a.32508].

108.   [DUPONT, Veronique. L'osteogenese imparfaite. Th: Pharma, 2004; P 4-
30, 100-104].

109.   [Thompson EM. Non-invasive prenatal dignosis of osteogenesis
imperfecta. Am J Med Genetics. 1993; 45: 201-6].

110.   [Berge LN, Marton V, Tranebjaerg L, Keamey MS, Kiserud T, Orian P.
Prenatal diagnosis of osteogenesis imperfecta. Acta Obstet Gynecol Scand 1995;
74: 321-3].

111.   [Redon JY, Gloaguen D, Collet M, Parent P, Le Grevellec JY. Osteogenesis
imperfecta. Reflections on prenatal diagnosis (about two cases). J Gynecol
Obstet Biol Reprod 1993; 22 :173 - 8].

112.   [Colet M, Le Guem H, Boog G. Diagnosis of limb malformations: limb
anomaly. In: Echographie des malformations fœtales. Gillet JY, Boog G, Dumez Y,
Nisand I, Valette C. Paris, Vigot 1990: 263-301].

113.   [Roger Valerie. Antenatal diagnosis of osteogenesis imperfecta. Th: Med:
Bordeaux II. 1997, P 51-97].

114.   [Kempe CH., Silverman FN., Steele BF., Droegemuller W., Silver HK.The
battered child syndrome. JAMA. 1984; 251: 3288-94].

115.   [Rauch F, traverse R, Norman NE, Taylor A, Glorieux FH. Deficient bone

formation in idiopathic juvenile osteoporosis: histomorphometric study of canelous iliac bone. J Bone Miner Res 2000; 15: 957-63].

116. [Bianchine JW, Briaard-Guillemot ML, Maroteaux P, Frezal J, Harrison HE. Generalized osteoporosis with bilateral pseudo-glioma-an autosomal recessive disorder of connective tissue: report of three families-review of the literature. Am J Hum Genet 2010; 86: 389-98].

117. [Gong Y, Slee RB, Fukai N, et al. LDL recptor-related protein 5 (LRP5) affects bone accural and eye development. Cell 2001; 107:513-23].

118. [Amor DJ, Savarirayan R, Schneider AS, Bankier A. New case of Col-Aarpenter syndrome. Am J Med Genet 2000 Jun 5; 92(4): 273-7. Andersen PE, Hauge M. V. Osteogenesis imperfecta: a genetic, radiological and epidemiological study. Clin Genet 1989; 36: 250-5].

119. [Bank RA, Robins SP, Wijmenga C, Breslau-Siderius LJ, Bardoel AF, Van Der SluijsHA₇ Pruijs HE, Tekoppele JM. 1999. Defective collagen crossling king in bone, but not in ligament or cartilage, in Bruck syndrome: indication for a bone-specific telopeptidelysys hydroxylase on chromosome 17. Proc Natl Acad Sci USA 96:1054 1058].

120. [Kutsumi K, Nojima T, Yamashiro K, Hatae Y, Isu K, Ubayama Y, Yamasaki S. Hyperplastic callus formation in both femurs in osteogenesis imperfect. Skeletal Radio, 1997; 26: 744-5].

121. [Rutkowski R, Resnick P, McMaster Jh - osteosarcoma occurring in osteogenesis imperfect: A case report. J Bone Joint Surg, 1979; 61B: 606-8].

122. [Manoj Ramachandran, MBBS, MRCS, FRCS. Osteogenesis Imperfecta Treatment & Management; Chief Editor: Harris Gellman, MD more. Nov 29, 2018]

123. [Caroline Marr, Alison Seasman, Nick Bishop. Managing the patients with osteogenesis imperfect: a multidisciplinary approach. Journal of Multidisciplinary Healthcare 2017: 10; 145-155]

124. [George Finidori. Constitutional diseases. Some orthopedic aspects. GEOP Gazette. Sep, Oct, Nov 2007. N°22: P, 10-17]

125. [Van Brussel & Engelbert - Physical training in children with osteogenesis imperfecta Journal of pediatrics, 2008]

126. [Schonau E. 10th international conference on osteogenesis imperfecta Ghent October 2008].

127. [Rauch F, Travers R, Parfitt AM, Glorieux FH. Static and dynamic bone histomorphometry in children with osteogenesis imperfecta. Bone 2000; 26: 581-9].

128.   [Glorieux FH, Bishop NJ, Polotkin H, Chabot G, Lanoue R, Travers R. Cyclic administration of panidronate in children with osteogenesis imperfecta. The New England journal of medicine 1998; 339: 947-952].

129.   [El Rakaawi-Hammoumraoui M, Djoudi H. Treatment with intravenous panidronate infusion during moderate to severe infantile osteogenesis imperfecta 2015.Thése de doctorat en médecine faculté de médecine de BLIDA].

130.   [Kutsumi K, Ayoob R, Bowden SA, Ingraham S, MahanJD. Beneficial effects of intravenous pamidronate treatment in children with osteogenesis imperfecta under 24 months of age. J Bone Miner Metab 2014; epub aheadof print].

131.   [Bishop N, Adami S, Ahmed SF, et al. Risedronate in children with osteogenesis imperfecta: A randomised, double-blind, placebo-controlled trial. Lancet 2013; 382:1424-32].

132.   [Carmel AS, Shieh A, Bang H, Bockman RS. The 25(OH)D level needed to maintain a favorable bisphosphonate response is M 33 ng/ml. Osteoporos Int 2012;23:2479-87].

133.   [Peris P, Martinez-Ferrer A, Monegal A, et al. 25 hydroxy vitamin D serum levels influence adequate response to bisphosphonate treatment in postmenopausal osteoporosis. Bone 2012; 51:54-8].

134.   [Munns CF, Rauche F, Zeitlin L, Fassier F, Glorieux FH. Delayed osteotomy but not fracture healing in pediatric osteogenesis imperfecta patient's recceving panidronate. J Bone Miner Res; 2004, 19(11): 1779-8176].

135.   [Whyte MP, McAlister WH, Novack DV, and Al. Biphosphonate-induced osteopetrosis: novel bone modeling defects, metaphyseal osteopenia and osteosclerosis fractures after drug exposure ceases. J Bone Miner Res 2008; 23: 1698 707].

136.   [K. Hachelaf, M. Amghar, B. RAFA, N. Dhiaf, O. Kerri, M.A. Benzemrane, A. Boumediene, F. Chouchaoui, A. Mekhaldi. Evaluation of the effect of the medical treatment "AREDEA - ZOMETA" on the consolidation of fractures or osteotomies of correction reinforced by telescopic pinning in osteogenesis imperfecta. Algerian Society of Rheumatology. 2016].

137.   [Grafe I, Yang T, Alexander S, et al. Excessive transforming growth factor-beta signaling is a common mechanism in osteogenesis imperfecta. Nat Med 2014; 20: 670-5].

138.   [Edwin M. Horwitz, Patricia L.Gordon, Winston K.k.Koo, Jeffrey C. Marx, Michael D.Neel, Rene Y McNall, Linda Muul, and Ted Hofmann. Isolated alloeneic

bone maroww-derive mesenchymal cells engraft and stimulate growth in children with osteogenesisimperfecta: implication for cell terapy of bone. PNAS. june 25,2002; n°13 vol 99, 8932-8937].

139.   [Ripkovic B, Anticevic D, Buljan M, Jakovina-Blazekovic S, Oreskovic Z, Kubat O. Characteristics of anesthesia in patients with osteogenesis imperfecta undergoing orthopedic surgical procedures. Lijec Vjesn. 2014 Sep-Oct; 136(9-10):291-5].

140.   [Olkestad L, Hald JD, Canudas-Romo V, Gram J, Hermann AP, Langdahl B, Abrahamsen B, Brixen K. Mortality and Causes of Death in Patients With Osteogenesis Imperfecta: A Register-Based Nationwide Cohort Study. J Bone Miner Res. 2016 Dec; 31(12):2159-2166].

141.   [Rebouilla J, Revelin P, Brault A. Surgical treatment of osteogenesis imperfecta by stepped osteotomies and diaphyseal pinning. Pédiatrie, 1969; 24: 411-20].

142.   [Baily RW, Dubow HI. Evolution of the concept of an extensible nail accommodating to normal longitudinal bone growth: Clinical consideration].

143.   [G. Finidori, Z. Pejin, V. Topouchian, C. Glorion. Fragile bones, palliative osteosynthesis. Bio-mechanical principles. La Gazette de la Société Française d'Orthopédie Pédiatrique. N°46. October - November 2016 : P : 11-12]

144.   [Mau H: In osteogenesis imperfecta no intra medullary nailing and especially no bone plates in child hood. Z Orthop ihre Grenzgeb, 1982, 120,297-308].

145.   [Chotigavanichaya C, Jadhav A, Bernstein RM, Watts HG: Rod diameter prediction in patiente with osteogenesis imperfect undergoing primary osteotomy. J Pediatr Ortho, 2001, 21,515-518].

146.   [Nicolas Nicolaou, John David Bowe, Mark Wilkinson. Use of Shiffield Telescopic Intramedullary Rod System for Management of Osteogehesis Imperfecta. Clinical Outcomes at an Average Follow-up of Nineteen Years. J Bone Joint Surg Am. 2011; 93: 1994-2000]

147.   [François Fassier. Telescopic nailing of the tibia in children. La Gazette de la société Française d'Orthopédie Pédiatrique. N°25. October-November 2008. P 14-17]

148.   [Fassier F and Al. Multicenter Radiological assessment of the Fassier-Duval femoral rodding, POSNA, San Diego 2006].

149.   [Azzam KA, Rush ET, Burke BR, Nabower AM, Esposito PW. Mid-term results of femoral and tibial osteotomies and Fassier-Duval nailing in children

with osteogenesis imperfecta. J Pediatr Orthop. Volume 38, Number 6, July 2018]

150.   [Tae-Joon Cho, MD, In Ho Choi, Chin Youb Chung, MD, Won Joon Yoo, MD, Ki Seok Lee, MD, and Dong yeon Lee, MD. Interlocking Telescopic Rod For Patients With Osteogenesis Imperfecta. Jour of Bone Joint Surg Am. 2007; 89:1028-35]

151.   [William Dias Belangero, Bruno Livani, Vera Maria, Santoro Belangero. Survival Rates of the HIMEX extensible nail in the treatment of children with osteogenesis imperfect. Acta Ortop Bras. 2010;18(6):343-8]

152.   [Hüseyin Günay, Levent Küçük, Muharrem İnan. The Results of the Treatment of Osteogenesis Imperfecta with Corkscrew Tipped Telescopic Nail. J Pediatr Res 2017; 4(1):17-20]

153.   [Boutaud B, Laville J-M. Centromedullary sliding pinning in osteogenesis imperfecta. Revue de Chirurgie Orthopédique. 2004 ; 90 : 304-311].

154.   [Hachelaf K, Dhiaf N, Benzemrane M.A, Kerri O, Guidoum Y, Mekhaldi A. Treatment of induced coxa vara of the femoral neck in osteogenesis imperfecta; apropos of 16 cases. Société Algérienne de chirurgie Orthopédique et traumatologique; Oral communication: Oran 2012]

155.   [P. Wicart, G. Finidori, Z. Pejin, C. Glorion. Congenital Coxa Vara in the hip of the child and adolescent. SOFOP monograph. Sauramps Medical. March 2017. P : 141-147]

156.   [Puvanesarajah V, Shapiro JR, principal sponsor. Sandwich allografts for long- bone nonunions in patients with osteogenesis imperfecta: a retrospective study. J Bone Joint Surg Am. 2015 Feb 18;97(4):318-25. doi: 10.2106/JBJS.N.00584]

157.   [N. Desai. Osteogenesis imperfecta and François Fassier. La Gazette de la SOFOP. N°46. October - November 2016: 6-8]

158.   [G. Finidori, M. Le Merrer, G. Pinto, V. Cormier Daire, G. Baujat, V. Topouchian, S.Pannier and Ch. Glorion. Note on the indications and administration protocols for biphosphates in children with osteogenesis imperfecta. La Gazette de la Société Française d'Orthopédie Pédiatrique. N°22. September-October-November 2007. P : 30]

159.   [G. Khalifa. LE SYSTEME EOS RADIOLOGIE NUMERIQUE BASSES DOSES. DESC de Chirurgie Pédiatrique. Session de mars 2009 - PARIS]

160.   [Hoffman DA, Lonstein JE, Morin MM. Breast cancer in women with scoliosis exposed to multiple diagnostic X rays. J Natl Cancer Inst 1989, 81: 1307-

1312]

161.   [Doody MM, Lonstein JE, Stovall M, Hacker DG, Luckyanov N, Land CE. Breast cancer mortality after diagnostic radiography: findings from the US Scoliosis Cohort Study. Spine 2000, 25: 2052-2063]

162.   [Hrubec Z, Boice JD, Monson RR, Rosenstein M. Breast Cancer after multiple chest fluoroscopies: second follow-up of Massachusetts Women with Tuberculosis. Cancer Res 1989, 49: 229-234]

163.   [Khalifa G, Charpak G, Maccia C, Fery-Lemonniere, BLOCH J, Boussard J.M, Attal M, Dubousset J, Amdamsbau C. - Evaluation of a new low-dose digital x-ray device: first dosimetric and clinical results in children. Pediatr Radiol 1998; 28: 557 61]

164.   [G. Khalifa. LE SYSTEME EOS RADIOLOGIE NUMERIQUE BASSES DOSES. DESC de Chirurgie Pédiatrique. Session de mars 2009 - PARIS]

165.   [J. Dubousset, G. Charpak, I. Dorion, W. Kalli, F. Lavaste, J. Deguise, G. Kalifa, S. Ferey. Le Système EOS. Nouvelle Imagerie Ostéo-Articulaire basse dose en position debout. e-mémoires de l'Académie Nationale de Chirurgie, 2005, 4 (4) : 22-27]

166.   [Mccall RE, Bax JA: Hyperplastic callus formation in osteogenesis imperfecta following intramedullary rodding. J Pediatr Orthop, 1984, 4, 361-364]

167.   [Mulpuri K, Joseph B: intramedullary rodding in osteogenesis imperfecta. J Pediatr Orthop, 2000, 20, 267-273]

168.   [P Lascombes, C Steiger, A Gonzalez, G de Coulon, R Dayer. Thirty-five years of stable elastic centromedullary embrochage (ECMES) in pediatric fractures: a method that is still young. e-mémoires de l'Académie Nationale de Chirurgie, 2015, 14 (1): 109-114]

169.   [Popkov , D. Use of flexible intramedullary nailing in combination with an external fixator for a postoperative defect and pseudarthrosis of femur in a girl with osteogenesis imperfecta type VIII: a case report. Strategies Trauma Limb Reconstr. 2018 Nov;13(3):191-197]

170.   [karbowski A, Schwitalle M, Brenner R, Lehmann H, Pontz B, Worsdorfer O: Experience With Bailly-Duboww Rodding in children with osteogenesisimperfecta.Eur J PeditrSurg, 2000, 10, 119-124]

171.   [James G. Gamble, M.D., Ph.D, Warren Jemes Strudwick, M.D., Lawrence, A. Rinsky, M.D., and Eugene E. Bieck, M.D. Complications of osteogenesis Imperfecta: Bailey-Dubow Rods Versus nonelongation Rods. Journal of Ped Orthop; 1988; 8: 645 649].

172.   [Lang-Stevenson AL, Sharrard W. intramedullary rodding with Billy Dubow extensible rods in osteogenesis imperfecta. An interim report of results and complications. J Bone Joint Surg(Br), 1984, 66, 227-32]

173.   [Janus Gj, Finidori G, Engelbert RH, Pouliquen M, Pruijs JE. Operative treatment of severe scoliosis in osteogenesis imperfecta/ results og 20 patents after halo traction and posterior spondylodesis with instrumentation. Eur Spine J. 2000 Dec; 9(6): 486-91]

174.   [Topouchian V, Finidori G, Glorion C, Padovani JP, Pouliqen JC. Posterior spinal fusion for kypho-scoliosis associated with osteogenesis imperfect: long-term results. Rev Chir Orthop Réparatrice App Mot. 2004 Oct ; 90(6) 525-32]

175.   [G. Finidori, V Topouchian, Z, Pejin, C Glorion. Surgical treatment of spinal deformities of osteogenesis imperfecta. La Gazette de la Société Française d'Orthopédie Pédiatrique. N° 46. October - November 2016. P : 14-18]

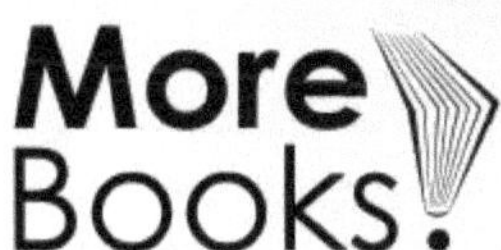

More
Books!

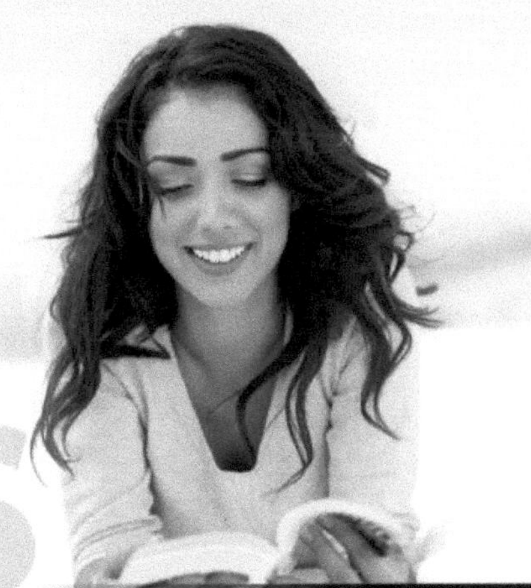

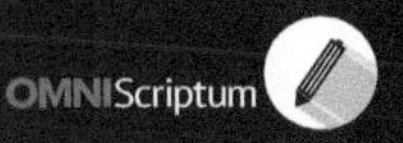

info@omniscriptum.com
www.omniscriptum.com
OMNIScriptum

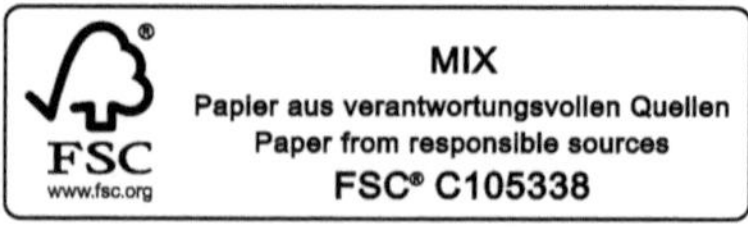

Printed by Books on Demand GmbH, Norderstedt / Germany